Advances in Transplant Dermatology

Fiona Zwald • Marc D. Brown
Editors

Advances in Transplant Dermatology

Clinical and Practical Implications

Springer

Editors
Fiona Zwald, MD, MCRPI
Transplant Dermatology
Piedmont Transplant Institute
Dermatology Consultants, PC
Atlanta
Georgia
USA

Marc D. Brown, MD
Department of Dermatology
University of Rochester
Rochester
New York
USA

ISBN 978-3-319-12444-5 ISBN 978-3-319-12445-2 (eBook)
DOI 10.1007/978-3-319-12445-2
Springer Cham Heidelberg New York Dordrecht London

Library of Congress Control Number: 2014958740

Printed on acid-free paper

Springer is part of Springer Science+Business Media (www.springer.com)

To my husband Jim, friend and loving partner who is a constant source of encouragement and support. To my two wonderful children Tara and Sara, a blessing and a joy. To my brother Philip, physician and scientist, for his perspective and brilliance. But most of all to our organ transplant patients, whose courage, hope and resilience is an inspiration to us all.

F. Zwald

To my family, my mentors, and my patients: you have made my career as a physician more rewarding than I ever imagined; thank you

M.D. Brown

Foreword

As the field of Transplant Dermatology moves through the second decade of truly collaborative, multinational activity, *Advances in Transplant Dermatology: Clinical and Practical Implications* represents a seminal consolidation of the current state of knowledge in this fascinating and complicated field. Substantial advancements in Transplant Dermatology have included changes in the immunosuppressant regimens that permit allograft survival; identification of novel viruses responsible for transplant-associated malignancies; increased understanding of benign and inflammatory skin disorders associated with transplant medications; advancements in the understanding of the impact of various forms of immunosuppression on the risk of cutaneous carcinogenesis and infections; broadening of the therapeutic repertoire available for the prevention and management of cutaneous malignancies; and, perhaps most importantly, substantial advancements in our understanding of optimal methods for staging and treating high-risk skin cancers in this vulnerable population. This volume presents the collective wisdom of world-class investigators in the field of Transplant Dermatology, elucidating these questions and more.

Dr. Fiona Zwald and Dr. Marc Brown are high-impact leaders in the field of Transplant Dermatology. Both having served as President of the International Transplant Skin Cancer Collaborative, an nonprofit organization dedicated to the advancement of knowledge related to transplant-related skin cancer, Drs. Zwald and Brown extend their long list of accomplishments and contributions to the field. Drs. Zwald and Brown have been instrumental in the organization of numerous educational meetings focused on Transplant Dermatology as well as being key contributors to data within the primary literature in the field. *Advances in Transplant Dermatology: Clinical and Practical Implications* represents a greatly needed update to the scholarly literature supporting the advancement of the field of Transplant Dermatology. We are all indebted to Drs. Zwald and Brown for coordinating and bringing together this outstanding compilation of the most up-to-date information in this complex and ever-changing field.

Rochester, MN, USA — Clark C. Otley, MD
Oklahoma, OK, USA — Thomas Stasko, MD

Preface

Solid organ transplantation represents a truly remarkable achievement in modern medicine, offering a new lease of life to many patients with terminal organ failure. Advances in the field, attributable to a refinement in immunosuppression protocols, improvements in surgical techniques and perioperative multidisciplinary care, have resulted in better survival outcomes for an increasing number of solid organ transplant recipients.

The dermatologist plays a pivotal role in the care, both pre- and post-transplantation, of the solid organ transplant recipient. Immunosuppression, necessary for transplant survival, has the unintended consequence of a host of dermatologic conditions, inflammatory, infectious and neoplastic, most important of which is the development of skin cancer. Skin cancer remains the most commonly diagnosed cancer among solid organ transplant recipients, comprising nearly 40 % of all post-transplant malignancies.

Transplant dermatology has grown into a new and exciting subspecialty of medicine. I gratefully acknowledge and appreciate the first textbook in this field, *Skin Disease in Organ Transplantation*, edited by Drs. Otley, Stasko, Murphy, Hirose and Chong and Mr. Michael Griffin. This publication, *Advances in Transplant Dermatology*, serves to educate the readership of advances in the field of transplant dermatology since its first publication in 2006. I gratefully acknowledge the hard work and dedication of the contributors of this textbook, many of whom are members of the International Transplant Skin Cancer Collaborative (ITSCC), an organization which has grown immeasurably over the last 10 years and whose efforts and collaborative nature deserve special mention.

Through the efforts of ITSCC and our multiple nondermatology colleagues and collaborators in transplant surgery, transplant nephrology, hepatology, pulmonology, cardiology, infectious disease, surgical and medical oncology, family medicine, paediatrics and psychiatry, together with transplant coordinators, nurses and social service providers, multiple transplant dermatology multidisciplinary clinics have emerged all around the country, dedicated to the care of the transplant recipient. We all function as a team of which dermatology is proud to be an integral part.

We hope that *Advances in Dermatology* will provide you with a resource for the latest developments in the field. The text opens with an update on benign and inflammatory skin disease secondary to transplant medication and follows with advances in photoprotection and our recent understanding of the role of HPV and immunosuppression in cutaneous squamous cell carcinoma.

Advances in the application of photodynamic therapy is discussed, followed by an analysis of our recent knowledge in the diagnosis, prevention and management of high-risk squamous cell carcinoma, Merkel cell carcinoma and melanoma in the transplant recipient.

We hope that you enjoy this textbook and that it may serve as a resource to transplant health care providers of all specialties worldwide. Many challenges still face us in the field of transplantation and transplant dermatology. Ongoing research efforts and collaboration will hopefully continue to improve outcomes in transplantation and also improve the quality of life of the transplant recipient afflicted with chronic dermatologic disease or high-risk skin cancer. We gratefully acknowledge our patients, who teach us everyday lessons in resilience, hope and the joy of a second chance of life.

President, ITSCC 2014-6

Atlanta, GA, USA — Fiona Zwald, MD, MCRPI
Rochester, NY, USA — Marc D. Brown, MD

Contents

Contributors

Sarah Arron, MD, PhD Department of Dermatology, University of California, San Francisco, San Francisco, CA, USA

Chantal C. Bachmann, MD Dermatologische Klinik, Universitätsspital Zürich, Zürich, Switzerland

Jan Nico Bouwes Bavinck, MD, PhD Department of Dermatology, Leiden University Medical Center, Leiden, The Netherlands

Marc D. Brown, MD Department of Dermatology, Strong Memorial Hospital/University of Rochester Medicine, Rochester, NY, USA

John A. Carucci, MD, PhD The Ronald O. Perelman Department of Dermatology, NYU Dermatological Surgical Associates, New York, NY, USA

Cameron Chesnut, MD Internal Medicine, Dermatologic Surgery, University of Washington School of Medicine, Spokane, WA, USA

Maurits N.C. de Koning, PhD Research and Development, DDl Diagnostic Laboratory, Rijswijk, Zuid Holland, The Netherlands

Joseph Diehl, MD Division of Dermatology, Department of Medicine, UCLA, Los Angeles, CA, USA

Mariet C. Feltkamp, MD, PhD Medical Microbiology, Leiden University Medical Center, Leiden, The Netherlands

Roel E. Genders, MD Department of Dermatology, Leiden University Medical Center, Leiden, The Netherlands

Günther F.L. Hofbauer, MD Dermatologische Klinik, Universitätsspital Zürich, Zürich, Switzerland

Joanna N. Hooten, MD Department of Dermatology, Duke University Medical Center, Durham, NC, USA

Stephanie Jeanne Martin, MD Division of Dermatology, UCLA, Los Angeles, CA, USA

Oonagh Molloy, MB, MICGP National Photobiology Unit, Department of Dermatology, Beaumont and Mater Misericordiae Hospital, Dublin, Ireland

Gillian M. Murphy, MD, FRCPI, FRCP, Edin National Photobiology Unit, Department of Dermatology, Beaumont and Mater Misericordiae Hospital, Dublin, Ireland

Sarah A. Myers, MD Department of Dermatology, Duke University Medical Center, Durham, NC, USA

Clark C. Otley, MD Department of Dermatology, Mayo Clinic Rochester; Rochester Methodist Hospital, Rochester, MN, USA

Elsemieke I. Plasmeijer, MD, PhD Department of Dermatology, Leiden University Medical Center, Leiden, The Netherlands

Koen D. Quint, MD, PhD Department of Dermatology, Leiden University Medical Center, Leiden, The Netherlands

Jason Michael Rizzo, BS, PhD Department of Biochemistry, SUNY Buffalo School of Medicine & Biomedical Sciences, Buffalo, NY, USA

Ashley G. Rubin, MD Division of Dermatology, Department of Medicine, University of California, San Diego, San Diego, CA, USA

Kathryn Serowka, MD Department of Dermatology, University of California – Irvine, Irvine, CA, USA

Teresa Soriano, MD Department of Medicine/Dermatology, UCLA School of Medicine, Los Angeles, CA, USA

Seaver L. Soon, MD Dermatology and Dermatologic Surgery, Scripps Clinic, La Jolla, CA, USA

Mary L. Stevenson, MD The Ronald O. Perelman Department of Dermatology, NYU Langone Medical Center, New York, NY, USA

Ashley Wysong, MD, MS Dermatology and Dermatologic Surgery, Scripps Clinic, La Jolla, CA, USA

Siegrid S. Yu, MD Department of Dermatology, University of California, San Francisco, San Francisco, CA, USA

Nathalie C. Zeitouni, MDCM, FRCPC Department of Dermatology, Roswell Park Cancer Institute, Buffalo, NY, USA

Fiona Zwald, MD, MRCPI Transplant Dermatology, Piedmont Transplant Institute, Dermatology Consultants, PC, Atlanta, GA, USA

1 Update on Benign and Inflammatory Skin Disease Secondary to Transplant Medication

Joanna N. Hooten and Sarah A. Myers

Contents

J.N. Hooten, MD • S.A. Myers, MD (✉)
Department of Dermatology, Duke University Medical Center, Durham, NC, USA
e-mail: joanna.hooten@duke.edu; sarah.myers@duke.edu

Abbreviations

APC	Antigen-presenting cell
AZA	Azathioprine
EGF	Epidermal growth factor
EGFRI	Epidermal growth factor receptor inhibitors
FKBP12	FK506-binding protein
GVH	Immune-mediated graft failure
HHV	Herpes virus
HPV	Human papillomavirus
HSV	Herpes simplexvirus
HUS	Hemolytic uremic syndrome
MAPK	The RAS-mitogen-activated protein kinase pathway
MC	Molluscum contagiosum
MM	Mycophenolate mofetil
mTOR	Mammalian target of rapamycin
NMSC	Nonmelanoma skin cancer
SD	Seborrheic dermatitis
SH	Sebaceous hyperplasia
SOTR	Solid organ transplant recipients

1.1 Introduction

Solid organ transplantation is the treatment of choice for many patients with organ failure. At the end of 2010, over 260,000 organ transplant recipients were alive in the United States. More than 25,000 new organs were transplanted in 2011, the majority of which were kidney (16,055), liver (5,805), lung (1,830), and heart (1,949) [1]. Over

F. Zwald, M.D. Brown (eds.), *Advances in Transplant Dermatology: Clinical and Practical Implications*,
DOI 10.1007/978-3-319-12445-2_1,

the past 20 years, the number of solid organ transplantations performed annually and the 5-year graft survival have increased, both in large part due to safer and more effective immunosuppressive medications. The demographics of organ transplant recipients have also evolved with more transplantations being performed in patients aged 65 years or older and in minority groups [1]. These data indicate that not only are more people living with an organ transplant but the transplanted population is increasing in diversity. Furthermore, skin disorders occur at a greater frequency in solid organ transplant recipients (SOTR) largely due to immunosuppressant medications, which are generally successful in their therapeutic effect of suppressing the immune system. However, immunodeficiency, along with direct toxic effects of many medications, often causes cutaneous disorders. A dermatologist should be aware of the changing demographics and unique therapeutic factors affecting this patient population.

1.2 Immunosuppressives: Mechanism of Action

T cells are the main drivers of immune-mediated graft failure (GVH) and are, the major target of immunosuppressant medications [2]. Clinical immunosuppression typically occurs in three phases: induction therapy, maintenance therapy, and therapy of an acute rejection.

Induction therapy is targeted at depleting T cells to prevent early, acute rejection. This therapy usually takes place in close proximity to transplantation, starting either during the intraoperative or immediately postoperative period, and is completed within the first 1–2 weeks after transplantation. The most commonly used induction agents are either antibodies that deplete T cells or IL-2 receptor antagonists that prevent T cell activation [3–5]. Induction therapy is not always used; in 2011, close to half of lung, liver, and heart transplant recipients did not receive induction therapy. However, over 80 % of kidney transplant recipients did receive induction, most commonly a T cell–depleting agent [1]. Induction therapy may cause prolonged T cell depletion, with increased risk for opportunistic infections, post-transplantation lymphoproliferative disorder, and possibly autoimmune disease.

Maintenance immunosuppressive agents are often life-long therapies [6]. Maintenance therapies generally work by interfering with one of the three signals required for T cell activation and proliferation. Signal 1 occurs through the interaction between an antigen-presenting cell (APC) and the CD-3 receptor on a T cell. Signal 2 occurs when a costimulatory complex is formed between CD80 and CD86 on the APC and CD28 on the T cell. Together, these two signals activate three signal transduction pathways: the calcium-calcineurin pathway, the RAS-mitogen-activated protein (MAP) kinase pathway, and the nuclear factor-κB pathway [7]. Once activated, these pathways stimulate the expression of numerous inflammatory mediators, including cytokines, in particular interleukin-2. Il-2 and other cytokines activate the "target of rapamycin" (mTOR) pathway that triggers cellular proliferation, which constitutes signal 3. B-cells can also be involved in alloimmune responses, if their receptors are engaged by antigen, through the production of alloantibody against donor HLA antigen [8, 9]. Five main classes of the most commonly used maintenance therapies are calcineurin inhibitors, co-stimulation blockers, mammalian target of rapamycin (mTOR) inhibitors, antiproliferatives, and corticosteroids [10]. Given the diverse pathways involved in alloimmunity, combination immunosuppressive therapy is usually required for successful suppression of alloimmune responses.

Since 1980, several significant advances toward more effective and less toxic maintenance immunosuppression have made transplantation more successful. In early transplant medicine, azathioprine (AZA), which inhibits purine synthesis, was used for maintenance immunosuppressive medication until cyclosporine largely replaced it in the early 1980s [11]. Cyclosporine was much more effective at reducing rejection rates and improving 1-year graft survival, which made transplantation more successful. Cyclosporine works by forming a complex with cyclophilin, inhibiting the calcineurin pathway and decreasing the synthesis of key cytokine genes that promote T cell activation and proliferation [6, 12]. Cyclosporine has many adverse effects including nephrotoxicity, hemolytic uremic syndrome (HUS), hypertension, hyperlipidemia, diabetes mellitus, gingival hyperplasia, hirsutism, and skin changes [13]. In the 1990s, tacrolimus, another calcineurin inhibitor, was introduced. Tacrolimus blocks the calcineurin pathway by binding FK506-binding protein (FKBP12), a more potent inhibitor of calcineurin than cyclosporine. Tacrolimus is more likely to cause DM than cyclosporine and can similarly cause nephrotoxicity and HUS but is less likely to cause hyperlipidemia, hypertension, and skin changes [14]. Today, tacrolimus is the most frequently used CNI in maintenance immunosuppression due to its superiority in preventing early acute rejections; however, patient survival, graft function, infection, malignancy, and blood pressure profiles are similar to cyclosporine [1, 15, 16].

The next significant advancement in maintenance immunosuppression occurred in the early 1990s with the introduction of mycophenolate mofetil (MM). MM inhibits purine synthesis by blocking inosine monophosphate dehydrogenase, leading to a decrease in lymphocyte proliferation. Although it acts similarly to AZA, its use in combination with CNIs led to improved patient and graft survival and decreased early and late allograft rejection [17, 18]. Furthermore, MM has a much better side-effect profile and requires less monitoring, which is why it has largely replaced AZA and is used in the majority of maintenance regimens today.

More recent advances in immunosuppression came with the introduction of mTOR inhibitors, sirolimus, and everolimus. These drugs are macrolide antibiotics that bind FKBP12 and inhibit cytokine (IL-2) activation of the mTOR pathway, blocking lymphocyte activation and proliferation. Although they bind FKBP12 as tacrolimus does, they function independently of the calcineurin pathway [19, 20]. Their principle adverse effects include hyperlipidemia, thrombocytopenia, and impaired wound healing, but they can also cause mouth ulcers and skin lesions [21]. Although they were initially developed to use as combination therapy with cyclosporine, they can also potentiate cyclosporine's adverse effects including nephrotoxicity and incidence of HUS and hypertension [22, 23]. Combination immunosuppression with tacrolimus and sirolimus has also resulted in more renal dysfunction and hypertension than tacrolimus plus MM [24, 25]. These features, along with minimal data to support net benefit over harm, have deterred the widespread use of mTOR inhibitors in maintenance immunosuppression [15]. Of note, mTOR inhibitors have anti-angiogenesis effects, which may benefit SOTR who develop de novo cancer (including skin cancer) or those who have a high risk of developing cancer [15, 26].

Belatacept, which blocks the co-stimulation of T cell (CD28) by APCs (CD80/86), has been recently approved for maintenance immunosuppression in renal transplant patients. Randomized, controlled trials comparing the efficacy of belatacept to cyclosporine demonstrated similar patient and graft survival, with better renal function compared with cyclosporine [27–30]. The unintended consequences of co-stimulation blockade have not been fully elucidated; therefore, whether belatacept replaces CNIs in maintenance immunosuppressive regimens remains to be seen [31].

In summary, the most frequently used combination immunosuppressive therapy is currently tacrolimus + MM +/− corticosteroids [15]. Lung and heart SOTR require the most immunosuppression, while liver transplant recipients often require less immunosuppression overall and tolerate early minimization therapy [1].

1.3 Skin Disease in SOTR

Aside from the kidney disease, hypertension, hyperlipidemia, diabetes mellitus, and HUS caused by immunosuppressant medications, skin disease, both benign and malignant, affects a large portion of STOR. Much research and focus has been placed on the marked increase in development of cutaneous malignancies; however, benign and inflammatory skin diseases are common in this population and can have a tremendous impact on quality of life and medication compliance. A broad spectrum of skin conditions affects SOTR, and many studies have estimated the prevalence of cutaneous manifestations in SOTR to range from 12.5 to 71 % [32–36]. Several factors affect the incidence of skin disease in SOTR including patient characteristics (age, gender), phototype, sun exposure, previous viral exposures, HLA typing [37–41], type of transplantation, level of immunosuppression, and specific medication regime. The type of skin disorders also changes with time, with cutaneous infections and inflammatory disorders predominating during the early years and premalignant and malignant lesions increasing in incidence concordantly with time from transplant [36, 37, 42, 43].

1.4 Cutaneous Infections

Overall, the most frequently encountered cutaneous infections in transplant recipients are superficial fungal infections and viral warts. However, modification of immunosuppression over time influences both the susceptibility to and prevalence of infections in SOTR. Overall immunosuppression is determined by the number, dose, duration, and sequence of immunosuppressive medications [42]. Within the first month after transplantation, the most frequently encountered cutaneous infections are nosocomial, including MRSA and wound- and catheter-associated infections, and reactivation of previously acquired infections. Less common infections include HSV and overgrowth of colonizers Aspergillus and pseudomonas [42]. Opportunistic infections are uncommon in the first postoperative month, which highlights the role that duration of immunosuppression has in the susceptibility to infection [44]. The intermediate period from 1 to 6 months post-transplant is the most risky for the development of opportunistic infections as patients are typically on high immunosuppressant doses.

1.5 Viral Infections

Given the suppression of T cell immunity and the role of T lymphocytes in combating viral pathogen [45], viral infections tend to predominate 1–6 months post-transplantation [42]. Antiviral prophylaxis has significantly decreased the incidence of herpes virus (HHV) infections that historically occurred between 1–6 months post-transplantation [46, 47]. However, reactivation of HHV represents a significant risk in this patient population and is important to diagnose and treat. The most common HHV infections in SOTR are herpes simplexviruses (HSV) types 1 and 2, cytomegalovirus, Epstein-Barr virus, HHV-6, HHV-7, and HHV-8, which is the causative agent of Kaposi Sarcoma [43, 48]. HSV infection is most commonly manifested through mucocutaneous lesions in the organ transplant population and must be distinguished between sirolimus-induced mucositis in the appropriate setting [43, 49]. The risk of HSV infection decreases 6 months after transplantation as immunosuppression is tapered. However, when lesions develop, they can be painful, persistent, and rarely disseminate to distant organs [50]. The most common treatments are acyclovir and valacyclovir, which can be used acutely and as suppressive therapy. Alternatives for acyclovir-resistant HSV include foscarnet, cidofovir, and trifluridine [51–54]. In patients with prolonged or high-dose immunosuppression, such as lung-transplantation recipients or those with frequent episodes of rejection, consideration should be given to chronic suppressive antiviral therapy. Moreover, given the increased incidence and impact on quality of life of viral infections, routine antiviral prophylaxis may be reasonable for the majority of SOTR.

After the sixth postoperative month, SOTR continue to be at high risk for developing community-acquired infections, and over time more indolent infections begin to develop, which are frequently caused by human papillomaviruses (HPV) [55–59]. In a recent prevalence study of renal transplant recipients, the most common cutaneous infection was viral warts, which was found in 38 % of patients and increased in frequency in concordance with duration from transplant. These results were consistent with several previous studies [8, 60–63]. HPV in SOTR can be challenging to treat and is an additional risk factor for NMSC, especially in this patient population [64]. Treatment can either be attempted through physical destruction (cryotherapy, curettage, laser) or topical therapies including salicylic acid, podophyllum, cantharidin, trichloroacetic acid, topical cidofovir, topical vitamin D, retinoids, or imiquimod [43, 65]. Imiquimod is not approved for use in transplant patients but has been shown to be very effective in enhancing cytokine production and indirectly stimulating T cell activity, thereby increasing patients' ability to effectively eliminate viral lesions [66–68]. Progressive or symptomatic disease may warrant systemic therapy such as intravenous cidofovir [69, 70]. Even with clearance, viral warts are a chronic condition and recurrence should be anticipated.

Less frequently, molluscum contagiosum (MC), a poxvirus that infects squamous epithelia [71, 72], has been shown to occur in nearly 7 % of pediatric SOTR [73], extensively in immunocompromised patients due to HIV, corticosteroid use, or chemotherapy [74]. Atypical presentations in SOTR have also been reported including multiple, giant MC lesions and MC folliculitis [75–77]. MC can be treated by surgically removing the umbilicated core, cryoablation, electrodessication, cantharidin, trichloroacetic acid, podophyllum, and topical tretinoin [43, 78]. For more extensive cases, topical imiquimod or cidofovir gel may be used [43, 79, 80]. Other rare viral infections include viral-associated trichodysplasia spinulosa and acquired epidermodysplasia verruciformis [81, 82].

1.6 Fungal Infections

Cutaneous fungal infections also occur frequently due to the suppression of cell-mediated immunity and, possibly, a reduction in the concentration of APC in the epidermis and can vary greatly in presentation [83]. In the early post-transplantation period, when immunosuppression is greatest, disseminated candidiasis and aspergillosis, both primary and secondary cutaneous resulting from invasive disease, are frequently seen but with institutional variability in incidence. Immunosuppressive doses also tend to be high 1–6 months post-transplantation, and patients continue to be at significant risk of developing an opportunistic deep fungal infection. Common mycoses include dimorphic fungi infections, zygomycoses, phaeohyphomycosis, hyalohyphomycosis, and cryptococcosis as well as continued risk from Candida and Aspergillus. Skin lesions range from nonerythematous papules, erythematous macules, papules and nodules (+/− necrosis), hemorrhagic bullae, abscesses, and cellulitis. Cutaneous fungal infections may occur in isolation or be a clue to underlying systemic infection. Early recognition of systemic infection is imperative given the potential mortality associated with disseminated disease [84, 85]. As clinical presentation is variable and relatively nonspecific, a high index of suspicion and early biopsies of skin lesions for histologic examination and culture are critical for diagnosis. Therapy usually requires systemic antifungal compounds including triazoles such as voriconazole and posaconazole, amphotericin B, and echinocandins such as caspofungin, micafungin, and anidulafungin, but surgical debridement/excision may be an adjunct in localized disease.

Overall, superficial fungal infections represent more common infections in SOTR. Mucocutaneous candidiasis is frequent, especially early in post-transplantation [86]. Nystatin or topical azoles are commonly used as effective treatments for superficial Candida infections. Dermatophyte infections often present atypically due to a lack of erythema that is normally produced by local inflammation [87]. Pityriasis versicolor has been identified as the most common fungal infection in SOTR in several studies [88–92] and can be treated with topical or oral medications, most commonly topical azole antifungals. In more involved cases, oral itraconazole can be very effective, but drug interactions with immunosuppressant medications must be considered and discussed with the transplant team [93]. Other frequent infections include chronic tinea pedis and onychomycosis, both of which are more common with chronic immunosuppression [59, 88–90, 94]. Oral terbinafine is the treatment of choice and has the benefit of little interaction with immunosuppressants, but liver function should be monitored during therapy [95]. Majocchi's granuloma is a deep dermal folliculitis caused by dermatophytes that tends to occur more frequently on the lower extremity in males who are on chronic (>36 months) immunosuppression [96, 97]. The causative agent of Majocchi's granuloma is most frequently *Trichophyton rubrum*, but other fungal species have also been isolated. Regardless of the causative agent, systemic therapy is often utilized, many times in conjunction with topical antifungals [96].

1.7 Common Inflammatory Disorders and Benign Tumors

Although several of the inflammatory dermatoses encountered in SOTR are due to drug effects, several conditions arise from an immunosuppressed state or hypersensitivity reaction, including folliculitis, drug rash, keratosis pilaris, hair loss of telogen effluvium type, sebaceous hyperplasia, seborrheic dermatitis (SD), acrochordons, porokeratosis, and seborrheic warts [59]. Several of these disorders, including keratosis pilaris and SH, have a similar prevalence in the non-transplant population and, therefore, may be unrelated to transplantation in some SOTR [98–100]. Skin tags have been shown to increase with age, duration from transplant, and BMI of SOTR, which may also be unrelated to transplantation [59]. Folliculitis has been reported in many SOTR, more frequently in early post-transplantation period, in males, and with cyclosporine use [35, 36, 59]. SD has been reported to occur in 9.5 % of renal transplant recipients [101], which is much higher than SD prevalence of 1–5 % reported in the normal adult population [102, 103]. However, SD occurs at a higher rate in other immunosuppressed populations such has HIV patients [104–106], patients with carcinomas of the upper respiratory and GI tracts associated with heavy alcohol and tobacco use [107], patients undergoing PUVA [108], and mountain guides with excessive sun exposure [109]. Although the precise etiology of SD is unclear, the commonality of immunosuppression in each of these populations suggests impaired T cell immunity leading to an altered immune response to Malassezia species and more prevalent SD [101]. Treatment with combination topical antifungals, steroids, or calcineurin inhibitors remains the most effect therapy for SD in SOTR [101].

Porokeratoses are thought to arise from abnormal clonal expansion of keratinocytes and, in SOTR, typically present as an isolated, annular plaque with central atrophy and a hyperkeratotic rim but can also present in superficial disseminated forms [110–113]. The incidence of porokeratoses in SOTR, from two population-based studies, is between 8 and 10.68 % [112, 114]. Immunosuppression has been suggested to play a role through impairment of immune surveillance by Langerhans cells [115], and the development of porokeratoses has been directly linked to the strength of immunosuppressive therapy [116–118]. The risk of malignant transformation of porokeratosis to SCC in the general population is approximately 7 %, which may be greater in SOTR secondary to immunosuppression, larger lesion sizes, and configuration [119]. Treatment of porokeratosis can present a challenge and is usually approached through topical chemotherapies including 5-fluorouracil or imiquimod, photodynamic therapy, and chemical peels; disseminated disease requires systemic therapy with oral retinoids [111].

Seborrheic warts are common in SOTR and, although their relationship with HPV status is unclear, a significant relationship between the quantity of seborrheic warts and NMSC, particularly BCC, has been established in SOTR [120]. Seborrheic warts are also more prevalent in lighter-skinned, older patients who had been transplanted the longest [120]. In patients with numerous seborrheic warts, acitretin can be helpful in decreasing lesion load [121].

1.8 Specific Drug-Induced Skin Changes: Immunosuppressants

1.8.1 Glucocorticoids

Aside from predisposing SOTR to infectious and inflammatory skin conditions, most immunosuppressive medications have direct toxic effects on the skin that vary with dose and duration of therapy. Historically, glucocorticoids were used at much higher doses compared with newer regimens; in fact, while many patients remain on chronic low doses, some immunosuppressive regimens have transitioned to steroid-free protocols [1]. The most frequent cutaneous complications of systemic steroids are acne, Cushingoid features, purpura, skin atrophy, and striae. Steroid-induced acne is dose-dependent and tends to present with monomorphic inflammatory papules and pustules on the trunk and upper extremities. This eruption is a neutrophilic folliculitis rather than true acne [122]. Treatment consists of decreasing the glucocorticoid dose and a trial of topical therapies including benzoyl peroxide, erythromycin, and clindamycin [123]. Oral therapies, including doxycycline and other oral antibiotics similarly used for acne, spironolactone in non-child-bearing women and isotretinoin, may be required for more resistant cases [85]. Glucocorticoids lead to redistribution of fat to the face, neck, and trunk characteristic of Cushingoid appearance, which is frequent in the immediate post-transplantation period when higher doses of systemic steroids are often used; as these doses are tapered, the Cushingoid features may or may not resolve. Purpura, related to skin atrophy, is also frequently seen in patients on long-term glucocorticoids and may be minimized using topical retinoids (0.01–0.05 %) or ammonium lactate (6–12 %) [85]. Striae, mainly located over the abdomen, thighs, and buttocks, may develop in patients on high-dose or long-term glucocorticoid therapy, particularly children and women. Striae are difficult to treat and no high-quality studies have found effective treatments [73, 124], but topical retinoids or pulsed dye laser may be helpful in early erythematous lesions [125, 126].

1.8.2 Cyclosporine

Cyclosporine has largely been replaced by more effective and safer immunosuppressant medications. Furthermore, the doses are lower than those historically used. These trends have decreased the frequency of cutaneous adverse effects, which tend to be dose-dependent. The most common cutaneous effects of cyclosporine include frequent hypertrichosis, possibly through increased activity of alpha reductase, leading to increased levels of dihydrotestosterone in peripheral tissues [127, 128]. Pilosebaceous lesions are also a common development as cyclosporine may be partially eliminated through sebaceous glands and pathogenic in folliculodystrophy [129]. Clinical lesions include sebaceous hyperplasia (SH), predominantly in male transplant patients; epidermal cysts; keratosis pilaris; and more nonspecific follicular eruptions [130–133]. Most of these conditions do not require intervention, but for extensive or irritated SH, intralesional desiccation [134], photodynamic therapy [135, 136], bichloracetic acid [137], and isotretinoin [138, 139] have been helpful in lesion reduction. Rarely, recalcitrant hyperplastic folliculitis and pilomatrix dysplasia have been reported [140–142]. Gingival hyperplasia is another well-known side effect, which occurs in approximately 1/3 of patients and generally begins after 3 months of therapy. It can be exacerbated by poor oral hygiene or concomitant use of phenytoin and calcium channel blockers [59, 85, 143]. Azithromycin may improve overgrowth and clinical appearance [144, 145].

1.8.3 Tacrolimus

Despite numerous potential systemic side effects, very few reports of cutaneous side effects related to tacrolimus have been published. Several cases of alopecia, more commonly occurring in females, have been reported and respond to either decreased dosage or alternative medication [146–148]. Interestingly, although topical tacrolimus is used in general dermatology for atopic dermatitis, tacrolimus-induced atopic dermatitis has been reported in rare cases when tacrolimus is used as a systemic immunosuppressant [149, 150]. Multiple epidermal cysts erupting in a patient on systemic tacrolimus has also been reported [151].

1.8.4 mTOR Inhibitors

Sirolimus and everolimus are immunosuppressive alternatives, especially in SOTR who develop numerous cutaneous squamous cell carcinomas. Sirolimus is more commonly used and associated with specific cutaneous side effects. The most frequent side effect is aphthous ulcerations, which can be severe [152–155]. Mucosal ulcerations occur more frequently with loading doses of sirolimus, which suggests a correlation between ulcerations and sirolimus dose. The ulcerations are largely self-limiting but can be a recurring problem [152]. When aphthae occur, ensuring the level of sirolimus is within the therapeutic range can be helpful. Aggressive use of potent topical steroids may also aid in resolution [152]. Pilosebaceous dermatoses also occur, most frequently presenting as an acne-like eruption within 1 month of starting sirolimus [49, 156–158]. These eruptions occur in nearly 50 % of patients, with a strong male predilection, and consist mostly of inflammatory papules, pustules, and occasional painful nodules involving the face and trunk [156, 157]. A possible mechanism for the pathogenesis of this inflammatory eruption is inhibition of the epidermal growth factor (EGF) pathway [159]. Topical therapy may be helpful, but systemic therapy with oral antibiotics is often required, and discontinuation of sirolimus may be necessary for recalcitrant cases [156, 158]. Leukocytoclastic vasculitis due to sirolimus therapy is rarer but also requires discontinuation of sirolimus [155, 160, 161]. Disorders of the nail, consisting of onycholysis, erythema, splinter hemorrhages, and pyogenic granulomas have also been reported with sirolimus [153]. Similar effects have been seen in patients transitioned to everolimus due to increased incidence of NMSC [162, 163].

1.8.5 Azathioprine

Minimal cutaneous adverse effects may be seen with AZA, mostly affecting the hair, including thinning of the hair or changes in hair color and texture [164, 165]. An erythema nodosum hypersensitivity reaction has also been reported in patients receiving AZA for inflammatory bowel disease, which may have been a result of the underlying illness rather than a direct effect of AZA [166].

1.8.6 Mycophenolate

The most frequent side effect related to MM is aphthous stomatitis, which can present more severely in patients who are on MM and mTOR inhibitors [152, 167]. Individual cases of dyshidrotic eczema and onycholysis attributed to MM have also been reported [168, 169].

1.9 Specific Drug-Induced Skin Changes: Other

Several non-immunosuppressant medications with cutaneous side effects may also be encountered during long-term care of transplant patients including retinoids, voriconazole, and epidermal growth factor receptor inhibitors (EGFRI).

1.9.1 Retinoids

Dermatologists caring for SOTR frequently encounter early onset and high tumor burden of NMSC and often utilize oral retinoids as a management strategy. Retinoids promote cellular differentiation, help control epithelial growth, downregulate proto-oncogenes, and can be a very effective chemoprevention for NMSC [170–172]. Adverse cutaneous effects of oral retinoid therapy are well documented, largely dose-dependent, and include mucocutaneous xerosis, the most common manifestations being cheilitis, generalized xerosis, palmoplantar desquamation, hair loss, nail dystrophy, eczema exacerbation, and skin fragility [170, 173, 174]. Initiating acitretin at 10 mg per day and increasing by 10 mg increments at 2–4 week intervals to desired effect helps minimize side effects and improve patient compliance [175].

1.9.2 Voriconazole

Voriconazole is frequently used as a prophylactic antifungal therapy and for the treatment of severe fungal infections, especially in lung transplant recipients. Voriconazole can have adverse cutaneous effects in up to 8 % of patients, with phototoxicity being reported most frequently, but cheilitis (often associated with phototoxicity), worsening of psoriasis, alopecia, and pruritus are also reported [176]. The clinical presentation and time course of voriconazole-induced phototoxicity are variable. Clinical lesions have been described as erythema, erythema plus cheilitis, erythema plus lentigines, erythema plus keratosis, bullous erythema, and pseudoporphyria. Regardless of the clinical presentation, the lesions are photodistributed, involving face, upper chest, arms, hands, and legs [176]. The photodistributed erythema and associated pigmentation changes suggest a phototoxic mechanism for the photosensitivity [177, 178]. A genetic polymorphism that decreases metabolism of voriconazole may also be involved in increasing photosensitivity in affected individuals [179].

Voriconazole phototoxicity is not a limited benign cutaneous reaction as several cases of squamous cell carcinoma as well as in situ melanoma arising within chronic phototoxic lesions, have been reported secondary to voriconazole photocarcinogenesis [180–183]. Patients who are prescribed voriconazole should be made aware of these risks and must be educated about the importance of aggressive photoprotection. In patients who develop phototoxicity, voriconazole should be substituted with an alternative antifungal, such as posaconazole. Physicians caring for SOTR should consider alternatives to voriconazole altogether in patients at high risk for skin cancer [184].

1.9.3 EGFRI

Skin cancer, in particular squamous cell carcinoma (SCC), is a well-known consequence of long-term immunosuppression [40, 185–187]. Epidermal growth factor receptor inhibitors (EGFRI) can block the proliferation of undifferentiated basal epidermal keratinocytes and, therefore, can be used as a targeted chemotherapy in head and neck squamous cell carcinomas [184, 188, 189]. EGFRI work either by targeting the extracellular EGFR domains (cetuximab and panitumumab) or by inhibiting the intracellular EGFR tyrosine kinase (erlotinib, gefitinib, and lapatinib) [190]. Such targeted therapies may provide a promising strategy for the treatment of patients with aggressive cutaneous SCC and are being investigated in clinical trials. Most common adverse effects with EGFR blockade are skin toxicities. Within the first 2–4 weeks of therapy, over 50 % of patients taking EGFRI develop a dose-dependent acneiform eruption, consisting of non-comedonal, erythematous papules and pustules that primarily involve the head, neck and upper trunk, and extremities [191, 192]. The eruption typically improves after reaching greatest activity within 3 weeks and, thus, discontinuation of the therapy is not usually required. In fact, the incidence and severity of the acneiform eruptions correlate with a better response to EGFRI therapy [193]. Xerosis is a common finding in patients on EGFRI therapy; therefore, moisturizing and mild cleansing of the skin are important. Other treatments include topical erythromycin, metronidazole, fusidic acid, zinc shake lotion, and doxycycline [193, 194]. Topical retinoids are not recommended because of their propensity to exacerbate dryness and irritation [195].

1.10 Summary

Management of cutaneous disorders in STOR involves both medical and surgical disciplines within dermatology. This population is at greater risk of cutaneous infections, inflammatory disorders, and skin cancer. Specialty dermatology clinics can be instrumental in addressing the increased incidence of skin disorders, both with diagnosis and treatment, when effective therapies exist. Informative counseling can also be of utmost importance in managing disease expectations and burden. Finally, when appropriate the dermatologist may have to recommend decreasing immunosuppressive therapy and should be able to determine the appropriate timing for this potential change. Functioning as part of the multidisciplinary team is of fundamental importance to successful management and outcomes for SOTR.

References

1. Organ Procurement and Transplantation Network (OPTN) and Scientific Registry of Transplant Recipients (SRTR). OPTN/SRTR 2011 Annual Data Report. Department of Health and Human Services, Health Resources and Services Administration, Healthcare Systems Bureau, Division of Transplantation; 2012. [11/5/2013]. Available from: http://srtr.transplant.hrsa.gov/annual_reports/2011/.
2. Rosenberg AS, Singer A. Cellular basis of skin allograft rejection: an in vivo model of immune-mediated tissue destruction. Annu Rev Immunol. 1992;10:333–58. PubMed PMID: 1590990. Epub 1992/01/01. eng.
3. Beiras-Fernandez A, Thein E, Hammer C. Induction of immunosuppression with polyclonal antithymocyte globulins: an overview. Exp Clin Transplant. 2003;1(2):79–84. PubMed PMID: 15859913. Epub 2005/04/30. eng.
4. Mottershead M, Neuberger J. Daclizumab. Expert Opin Biol Ther. 2007;7(10):1583–96. PubMed PMID: 17916050. Epub 2007/10/06. eng.
5. Ramirez CB, Marino IR. The role of basiliximab induction therapy in organ transplantation. Expert Opin Biol Ther. 2007;7(1):137–48. PubMed PMID: 17150025. Epub 2006/12/08. eng.
6. Halloran PF. Immunosuppressive drugs for kidney transplantation. N Engl J Med. 2004;351(26):2715–29. PubMed PMID: 15616206. Epub 2004/12/24. eng.
7. Wang D, Matsumoto R, You Y, Che T, Lin XY, Gaffen SL, et al. CD3/CD28 costimulation-induced NF-kappaB activation is mediated by recruitment of protein kinase C-theta, Bcl10, and IkappaB kinase beta to the immunological synapse through CARMA1. Mol Cell Biol. 2004;24(1):164–71. PubMed PMID: 14673152. Pubmed Central PMCID: PMC303359. Epub 2003/12/16. eng.
8. MacLennan IC, Toellner KM, Cunningham AF, Serre K, Sze DM, Zuniga E, et al. Extrafollicular antibody responses. Immunol Rev. 2003;194:8–18. PubMed PMID: 12846803. Epub 2003/07/09. eng.
9. Sarwal M, Chua MS, Kambham N, Hsieh SC, Satterwhite T, Masek M, et al. Molecular heterogeneity in acute renal allograft rejection identified by DNA microarray profiling. N Engl J Med. 2003;349(2):125–38. PubMed PMID: 12853585. Epub 2003/07/11. eng.
10. Lee RA, Gabardi S. Current trends in immunosuppressive therapies for renal transplant recipients. Am J Health Syst Pharm. 2012;69(22):1961–75. PubMed PMID: 23135563. Epub 2012/11/09. eng.
11. Elion GB. The George Hitchings and Gertrude Elion Lecture. The pharmacology of azathioprine. Ann N Y Acad Sci. 1993;685:400–7. PubMed PMID: 8363248. Epub 1993/06/23. eng.
12. Hardinger KL, Koch MJ, Brennan DC. Current and future immunosuppressive strategies in renal transplantation. Pharmacotherapy. 2004;24(9):1159–76. PubMed PMID: 15460177. Epub 2004/10/06. eng.
13. Sandimmune (cyclosporine) [package insert]. East Hanover: Novartis Pharmaceuticals Corporation; 2013.
14. Prograf (tacrolimus) [package insert]. Deerfield: Astellas Pharma US; 2013.
15. KDIGO Transplant Work Group. KDIGO clinical practice guideline for the care of kidney transplant recipients. Am J Transplant. 2009;9 Suppl 3:S1–155. PubMed PMID: 19845597. Epub 2009/10/23. eng.
16. Bia M, Adey DB, Bloom RD, Chan L, Kulkarni S, Tomlanovich S. KDOQI US commentary on the 2009 KDIGO clinical practice guideline for the care of kidney transplant recipients. Am J Kidney Dis. 2010;56(2):189–218. PubMed PMID: 20598411. Epub 2010/07/06. eng.
17. Meier-Kriesche HU, Steffen BJ, Hochberg AM, Gordon RD, Liebman MN, Morris JA, et al. Mycophenolate mofetil versus azathioprine therapy is associated with a significant protection against long-term renal allograft function deterioration. Transplantation. 2003;75(8):1341–6. PubMed PMID: 12717227. Epub 2003/04/30. eng.
18. Gourishankar S, Hunsicker LG, Jhangri GS, Cockfield SM, Halloran PF. The stability of the glomerular filtration rate after renal transplantation is improving. J Am Soc Nephrol. 2003;14(9):2387–94. PubMed PMID: 12937318. Epub 2003/08/26. eng.
19. Abraham RT, Wiederrecht GJ. Immunopharmacology of rapamycin. Annu Rev Immunol. 1996;14:483–510. PubMed PMID: 8717522. Epub 1996/01/01. eng.
20. Bierer BE, Mattila PS, Standaert RF, Herzenberg LA, Burakoff SJ, Crabtree G, et al. Two distinct signal transmission pathways in T lymphocytes are inhibited by complexes formed between an immunophilin and either FK506 or rapamycin. Proc Natl Acad Sci U S A. 1990;87(23):9231–5. PubMed PMID: 2123553. Pubmed Central PMCID: PMC55138. Epub 1990/12/01. eng.
21. Rapamune (sirolimus) [package insert]. Philadelphia: Wyeth Pharmaceuticals Inc, a subsidiary of Pfizer Inc.
22. MacDonald AS. A worldwide, phase III, randomized, controlled, safety and efficacy study of a sirolimus/cyclosporine regimen for prevention of acute rejection in recipients of primary mismatched renal allografts. Transplantation. 2001;71(2):271–80. PubMed PMID: 11213073. Epub 2001/02/24. eng.
23. Kahan BD. Efficacy of sirolimus compared with azathioprine for reduction of acute renal allograft rejection: a randomised multicentre study. The Rapamune US Study Group. Lancet. 2000;356(9225):194–202. PubMed PMID: 10963197. Epub 2000/08/30. eng.
24. McAlister VC, Gao Z, Peltekian K, Domingues J, Mahalati K, MacDonald AS. Sirolimus-tacrolimus combination immunosuppression. Lancet. 2000;355(9201):376–7. PubMed PMID: 10665560. Epub 2000/02/09. eng.
25. Gonwa T, Mendez R, Yang HC, Weinstein S, Jensik S, Steinberg S. Randomized trial of tacrolimus

in combination with sirolimus or mycophenolate mofetil in kidney transplantation: results at 6 months. Transplantation. 2003;75(8):1213–20. PubMed PMID: 12717205. Epub 2003/04/30. eng.
26. Gabardi S, Baroletti SA. Everolimus: a proliferation signal inhibitor with clinical applications in organ transplantation, oncology, and cardiology. Pharmacotherapy. 2010;30(10):1044–56. PubMed PMID: 20874042. Epub 2010/09/30. eng.
27. Rostaing L, Vincenti F, Grinyo J, Rice KM, Bresnahan B, Steinberg S, et al. Long-term belatacept exposure maintains efficacy and safety at 5 years: results from the long-term extension of the BENEFIT study. Am J Transplant. 2013;13(11):2875–83. PubMed PMID: 24047110. Epub 2013/09/21. eng.
28. Grinyo J, Alberu J, Contieri FL, Manfro RC, Mondragon G, Nainan G, et al. Improvement in renal function in kidney transplant recipients switched from cyclosporine or tacrolimus to belatacept: 2-year results from the long-term extension of a phase II study. Transpl Int. 2012;25(10):1059–64. PubMed PMID: 22816557. Epub 2012/07/24. eng.
29. Pestana JO, Grinyo JM, Vanrenterghem Y, Becker T, Campistol JM, Florman S, et al. Three-year outcomes from BENEFIT-EXT: a phase III study of belatacept versus cyclosporine in recipients of extended criteria donor kidneys. Am J Transplant. 2012;12(3):630–9. PubMed PMID: 22300431. Epub 2012/02/04. eng.
30. Rostaing L, Massari P, Garcia VD, Mancilla-Urrea E, Nainan G, del Carmen Rial M, et al. Switching from calcineurin inhibitor-based regimens to a belatacept-based regimen in renal transplant recipients: a randomized phase II study. Clin J Am Soc Nephrol. 2011;6(2):430–9. PubMed PMID: 21051752. Pubmed Central PMCID: PMC3052236. Epub 2010/11/06. eng.
31. Riella LV, Sayegh MH. T-cell co-stimulatory blockade in transplantation: two steps forward one step back! Expert Opin Biol Ther. 2013;13(11):1557–68. PubMed PMID: 24083381. Epub 2013/10/03. eng.
32. Formicone F, Fargnoli MC, Pisani F, Rascente M, Famulari A, Peris K. Cutaneous manifestations in Italian kidney transplant recipients. Transplant Proc. 2005;37(6):2527–8. PubMed PMID: 16182734. Epub 2005/09/27. eng.
33. Hassan G, Khalaf H, Mourad W. Dermatologic complications after liver transplantation: a single-center experience. Transplant Proc. 2007;39(4):1190–4. PubMed PMID: 175249290. Epub 2007/05/26. eng.
34. Perera GK, Child FJ, Heaton N, O'Grady J, Higgins EM. Skin lesions in adult liver transplant recipients: a study of 100 consecutive patients. Br J Dermatol. 2006;154(5):868–72. PubMed PMID: 16634888. Epub 2006/04/26. eng.
35. Belloni-Fortina A, Piaserico S, Bordignon M, Gambato M, Senzolo M, Russo FP, et al. Skin cancer and other cutaneous disorders in liver transplant recipients. Acta Derm Venereol. 2012;92(4):411–5. PubMed PMID: 22377797. Epub 2012/03/02. eng.
36. Wisgerhof HC, Edelbroek JR, de Fijter JW, Feltkamp MC, Willemze R, Bouwes Bavinck JN. Trends of skin diseases in organ-transplant recipients transplanted between 1966 and 2006: a cohort study with follow-up between 1994 and 2006. Br J Dermatol. 2010;162(2):390–6. PubMed PMID: 19799604. Epub 2009/10/06. eng.
37. Bouwes Bavinck JN, Kootte AM, Van Der Woude FJ, Vandenbroucke JP, Vermeer BJ, Claas FH. On a possible protective effect of HLA-A11 against skin cancer and keratotic skin lesions in renal transplant recipients. J Invest Dermatol. 1991;97(2):269–72. PubMed PMID: 1649229. Epub 1991/08/01. eng.
38. Streilein JW. Immunogenetic factors in skin cancer. N Engl J Med. 1991;325(12):884–7. PubMed PMID: 1875975. Epub 1991/09/19. eng.
39. Mithoefer AB, Supran S, Freeman RB. Risk factors associated with the development of skin cancer after liver transplantation. Liver Transpl. 2002;8(10):939–44. PubMed PMID: 12360438. Epub 2002/10/03. eng.
40. Mudigonda T, Levender MM, O'Neill JL, West CE, Pearce DJ, Feldman SR. Incidence, risk factors, and preventative management of skin cancers in organ transplant recipients: a review of single- and multicenter retrospective studies from 2006 to 2010. Dermatol Surg. 2013;39(3 Pt 1):345–64. PubMed PMID: 23190408. Epub 2012/11/30. eng.
41. Gogia R, Binstock M, Hirose R, Boscardin WJ, Chren MM, Arron ST. Fitzpatrick skin phototype is an independent predictor of squamous cell carcinoma risk after solid organ transplantation. J Am Acad Dermatol. 2013;68(4):585–91. PubMed PMID: 23107311. Pubmed Central PMCID: PMC3562416. Epub 2012/10/31. eng.
42. Fishman JA. Infection in solid-organ transplant recipients. N Engl J Med. 2007;357(25):2601–14. PubMed PMID: 18094380. Epub 2007/12/21. eng.
43. Tan HH, Goh CL. Viral infections affecting the skin in organ transplant recipients: epidemiology and current management strategies. Am J Clin Dermatol. 2006;7(1):13–29. PubMed PMID: 16489840. Epub 2006/02/24. eng.
44. Rubin RH. Infectious disease complications of renal transplantation. Kidney Int. 1993;44(1):221–36. PubMed PMID: 8394951. Epub 1993/07/01. eng.
45. Baron S. Medical microbiology. 4th ed. Galveston: University of Texas Medical Branch; 1996.
46. Rubin RH, Kemmerly SA, Conti D, Doran M, Murray BM, Neylan JF, et al. Prevention of primary cytomegalovirus disease in organ transplant recipients with oral ganciclovir or oral acyclovir prophylaxis. Transpl Infect Dis. 2000;2(3):112–7. PubMed PMID: 11429021. Epub 2001/06/29. eng.
47. Meyers JD, Wade JC, Mitchell CD, Saral R, Lietman PS, Durack DT, et al. Multicenter collaborative trial of intravenous acyclovir for treatment of mucocutaneous herpes simplex virus infection in the immunocompromised host. Am J Med. 1982;73(1A):229–35. PubMed PMID: 7048914. Epub 1982/07/20. eng.
48. Griffiths WJ, Wreghitt TG, Alexander GJ. Reactivation of herpes simplex virus after liver transplantation.

Transplantation. 2005;80(9):1353–4. PubMed PMID: 16314807. Epub 2005/11/30. eng.
49. Montalbano M, Neff GW, Yamashiki N, Meyer D, Bettiol M, Slapak-Green G, et al. A retrospective review of liver transplant patients treated with sirolimus from a single center: an analysis of sirolimus-related complications. Transplantation. 2004;78(2):264–8. PubMed PMID: 15280688. Epub 2004/07/29. eng.
50. Smith SR, Butterly DW, Alexander BD, Greenberg A. Viral infections after renal transplantation. Am J Kidney Dis. 2001;37(4):659–76. PubMed PMID: 11273865. Epub 2001/03/29. eng.
51. Mendel DB, Barkhimer DB, Chen MS. Biochemical basis for increased susceptibility to Cidofovir of herpes simplex viruses with altered or deficient thymidine kinase activity. Antimicrob Agents Chemother. 1995;39(9):2120–2. PubMed PMID: 8540727. Pubmed Central PMCID: PMC162892. Epub 1995/09/01. eng.
52. Chilukuri S, Rosen T. Management of acyclovir-resistant herpes simplex virus. Dermatol Clin. 2003;21(2):311–20. PubMed PMID: 12757254. Epub 2003/05/22. eng.
53. Vere Hodge RA, Field HJ. Antiviral agents for herpes simplex virus. Adv Pharmacol. 2013;67:1–38. PubMed PMID: 23885997. Epub 2013/07/28. eng.
54. Kessler HA, Hurwitz S, Farthing C, Benson CA, Feinberg J, Kuritzkes DR, et al. Pilot study of topical trifluridine for the treatment of acyclovir-resistant mucocutaneous herpes simplex disease in patients with AIDS (ACTG 172). AIDS Clinical Trials Group. J Acquir Immune Defic Syndr Hum Retrovirol. 1996;12(2):147–52. PubMed PMID: 8680885. Epub 1996/06/01. eng.
55. Fishman JA, Rubin RH. Infection in organ-transplant recipients. N Engl J Med. 1998;338(24):1741–51. PubMed PMID: 962419. 5. Epub 1998/06/12. eng.
56. Hogewoning AA, Goettsch W, van Loveren H, de Fijter JW, Vermeer BJ, Bouwes Bavinck JN. Skin infections in renal transplant recipients. Clin Transplant. 2001;15(1):32–8. PubMed PMID: 11168313. Epub 2001/02/13. eng.
57. Berkhout RJ, Bouwes Bavinck JN, ter Schegget J. Persistence of human papillomavirus DNA in benign and (pre)malignant skin lesions from renal transplant recipients. J Clin Microbiol. 2000;38(6):2087–96. PubMed PMID: 10834958. Pubmed Central PMCID: PMC86734. Epub 2000/06/02. eng.
58. de Jong-Tieben LM, Berkhout RJ, ter Schegget J, Vermeer BJ, de Fijter JW, Bruijn JA, et al. The prevalence of human papillomavirus DNA in benign keratotic skin lesions of renal transplant recipients with and without a history of skin cancer is equally high: a clinical study to assess risk factors for keratotic skin lesions and skin cancer. Transplantation. 2000;69(1):44–9. PubMed PMID: 10653378. Epub 2000/02/01. eng.
59. Lally A, Casabonne D, Imko-Walczuk B, Newton R, Wojnarowska F. Prevalence of benign cutaneous disease among Oxford renal transplant recipients. J Eur Acad Dermatol Venereol. 2011;25(4):462–70. PubMed PMID: 20738465. Epub 2010/08/27. eng.
60. Bouwes Bavinck JN, Berkhout RJ. HPV infections and immunosuppression. Clin Dermatol. 1997;15(3):427–37. PubMed PMID: 9255448. Epub 1997/05/01. eng.
61. de Lima AM, da Rocha SP, Reis Filho EG, Eid DR, Reis CM. Study of dermatoses in kidney transplant patients. An Bras Dermatol. 2013;88(3):361–7. PubMed PMID: 23793196. Pubmed Central PMCID: PMC3754366. Epub 2013/06/26. eng.
62. Rudlinger R, Smith IW, Bunney MH, Hunter JA. Human papillomavirus infections in a group of renal transplant recipients. Br J Dermatol. 1986;115(6):681–92. PubMed PMID: 3026431. Epub 1986/12/01. eng.
63. Blohme I, Larko O. Skin lesions in renal transplant patients after 10–23 years of immunosuppressive therapy. Acta Derm Venereol. 1990;70(6):491–4. PubMed PMID: 1981421. Epub 1990/01/01. eng.
64. Benton EC, McLaren K, Barr BB, Blessing K, Bunney MH, Rudlinger R, et al. Human papilloma virus infection and its relationship to skin cancer in a group of renal allograft recipients. Curr Probl Dermatol. 1989;18:168–77. PubMed PMID: 2545416. Epub 1989/01/01. eng.
65. Moscarelli L, Annunziata F, Mjeshtri A, Paudice N, Tsalouchos A, Zanazzi M, et al. Successful treatment of refractory wart with a topical activated vitamin d in a renal transplant recipient. Case Rep Transplant. 2011;2011:368623. PubMed PMID: 23198256. Pubmed Central PMCID: PMC3504230. Epub 2011/01/01. eng.
66. Miller RL, Gerster JF, Owens ML, Slade HB, Tomai MA. Imiquimod applied topically: a novel immune response modifier and new class of drug. Int J Immunopharmacol. 1999;21(1):1–14. PubMed PMID: 10411278. Epub 1999/07/20. eng.
67. Sauder DN. Immunomodulatory and pharmacologic properties of imiquimod. J Am Acad Dermatol. 2000;43(1 Pt 2):S6–11. PubMed PMID: 10861101. Epub 2000/06/22. eng.
68. Harwood CA, Perrett CM, Brown VL, Leigh IM, McGregor JM, Proby CM. Imiquimod cream 5 % for recalcitrant cutaneous warts in immunosuppressed individuals. Br J Dermatol. 2005;152(1):122–9.
69. Cusack C, Fitzgerald D, Clayton TM, Irvine AD. Successful treatment of florid cutaneous warts with intravenous cidofovir in an 11-year-old girl. Pediatr Dermatol. 2008;25(3):387–9.
70. Kottke MD, Parker SRS. Intravenous cidofovir-induced resolution of disfiguring cutaneous human papillomavirus infection. J Am Acad Dermatol. 2006;55(3):533–6.
71. Gottlieb SL, Myskowski PL. Molluscum contagiosum. Int J Dermatol. 1994;33(7):453–61. PubMed PMID: 7928025. Epub 1994/07/01. eng.
72. Waugh MA. Molluscum contagiosum. Dermatol Clin. 1998;16(4):839–41, xv. PubMed PMID: 9891691. Epub 1999/01/19. eng.
73. Euvrard S, Kanitakis J, Cochat P, Cambazard F, Claudy A. Skin diseases in children with organ transplants. J Am Acad Dermatol. 2001;44(6):932–9. PubMed PMID: 11369903. Epub 2001/05/23. eng.
74. Schwartz JJ, Myskowski PL. Molluscum contagiosum in patients with human immunodeficiency virus

infection. A review of twenty-seven patients. J Am Acad Dermatol. 1992;27(4):583–8. PubMed PMID: 1357010. Epub 1992/10/01. eng.

75. Gardner LS, Ormond PJ. Treatment of multiple giant molluscum contagiosum in a renal transplant patient with imiquimod 5 % cream. Clin Exp Dermatol. 2006;31(3):452–3. PubMed PMID: 16681599. Epub 2006/05/10. eng.
76. Mansur AT, Goktay F, Gunduz S, Serdar ZA. Multiple giant molluscum contagiosum in a renal transplant recipient. Transpl Infect Dis. 2004;6(3):120–3. PubMed PMID: 15569228. Epub 2004/12/01. eng.
77. Feldmeyer L, Kamarashev J, Boehler A, Irani S, Speich R, French LE, et al. Molluscum contagiosum folliculitis mimicking tinea barbae in a lung transplant recipient. J Am Acad Dermatol. 2010;63(1):169–71. PubMed PMID: 20542185. Epub 2010/06/15. eng.
78. Hanna D, Hatami A, Powell J, Marcoux D, Maari C, Savard P, et al. A prospective randomized trial comparing the efficacy and adverse effects of four recognized treatments of molluscum contagiosum in children. Pediatr Dermatol. 2006;23(6):574–9. PubMed PMID: 17156002. Epub 2006/12/13. eng.
79. Yazdani S, Stiehm ER. Topical imiquimod for molluscum contagiosum in T cell immunodeficiency. Pediatr Infect Dis J. 2003;22(6):575–6. PubMed PMID: 12799517. Epub 2010/06/15. eng.
80. Guerin M, Lepecheur V, Rachieru-Sourisseau P, Reguerre Y, Pellier I, Martin L. Usefulness of topical cidofovir treatment for recalcitrant molluscum contagiosum in immunocompromised children. Arch Pediatr. 2012;19(11):1157–63. PubMed PMID: 23037586. Epub 2012/10/06. Utilite du cidofovir topique dans le traitement des molluscums contagiosums en contexte d'immunosuppression therapeutique chez l'enfant. fre.
81. Gomez-Bernal S, Rodriguez-Pazos L, Pereiro-Ferreiros MM, Toribio J. Acquired epidermodysplasia verruciformis in a renal transplant recipient. Actas Dermosifiliogr. 2011;102(2):159–61. PubMed PMID: 21292228. Epub 2011/02/05. Epidermodisplasia verruciforme adquirida en una paciente transplantada renal. spa.
82. Sperling LC, Tomaszewski MM, Thomas DA. Viral-associated trichodysplasia in patients who are immunocompromised. J Am Acad Dermatol. 2004;50(2):318–22. PubMed PMID: 14726896. Epub 2004/01/17. eng.
83. Bergfelt L, Larko O, Blohme I. Skin disease in immunosuppressed patients in relation to epidermal Langerhans' cells. Acta Derm Venereol. 1993;73(5):330–4. PubMed PMID: 7904395. Epub 1993/10/01. eng.
84. Virgili A, Zampino MR, Mantovani L. Fungal skin infections in organ transplant recipients. Am J Clin Dermatol. 2002;3(1):19–35. PubMed PMID: 11817966. Epub 2002/01/31. eng.
85. Ponticelli C, Bencini PL. Nonneoplastic mucocutaneous lesions in organ transplant recipients. Transpl Int. 2011;24(11):1041–50. PubMed PMID: 21806688. Epub 2011/08/03. eng.
86. Ribeiro PM, Bacal F, Koga-Ito CY, Junqueira JC, Jorge AO. Presence of Candida spp. in the oral cavity of heart transplantation patients. J Appl Oral Sci. 2011;19(1):6–10. PubMed PMID: 21437462. Epub 2011/03/26. eng.
87. Miele PS, Levy CS, Smith MA, Dugan EM, Cooke RH, Light JA, et al. Primary cutaneous fungal infections in solid organ transplantation: a case series. Am J Transplant. 2002;2(7):678–83. PubMed PMID: 12201372. Epub 2002/08/31. eng.
88. Shuttleworth D, Philpot CM, Salaman JR. Cutaneous fungal infection following renal transplantation: a case control study. Br J Dermatol. 1987;117(5):585–90. PubMed PMID: 3318908. Epub 1987/11/01. eng.
89. Virgili A, Zampino MR, La Malfa V, Strumia R, Bedani PL. Prevalence of superficial dermatomycoses in 73 renal transplant recipients. Dermatology. 1999;199(1):31–4. PubMed PMID: 10449954. Epub 1999/08/18. eng.
90. Gulec AT, Demirbilek M, Seckin D, Can F, Saray Y, Sarifakioglu E, et al. Superficial fungal infections in 102 renal transplant recipients: a case–control study. J Am Acad Dermatol. 2003;49(2):187–92. PubMed PMID: 12894063. Epub 2003/08/02. eng.
91. Koranda FC, Dehmel EM, Kahn G, Penn I. Cutaneous complications in immunosuppressed renal homograft recipients. JAMA. 1974;229(4):419–24. PubMed PMID: 4275980. Epub 1974/07/22. eng.
92. Barba A, Tessari G, Boschiero L, Chieregato GC. Renal transplantation and skin diseases: review of the literature and results of a 5-year follow-up of 285 patients. Nephron. 1996;73(2):131–6. PubMed PMID: 8773333. Epub 1996/01/01. eng.
93. Hickman JG. A double-blind, randomized, placebo-controlled evaluation of short-term treatment with oral itraconazole in patients with tinea versicolor. J Am Acad Dermatol. 1996;34(5, Part 1):785–7.
94. Ray TL. Fungal infections in the immunocompromised host. Med Clin North Am. 1980;64(5):955–68. PubMed PMID: 7432049. Epub 1980/09/01. eng.
95. Ghannoum MA, Welshenbaugh A, Imamura Y, Isham N, Mallefet P, Yamaguchi H. Comparison of the in vitro activity of terbinafine and lanoconazole against dermatophytes. Mycoses. 2010;53(4):311–3. PubMed PMID: 19422522. Epub 2009/05/09. eng.
96. Romero FA, Deziel PJ, Razonable RR. Majocchi's granuloma in solid organ transplant recipients. Transpl Infect Dis. 2011;13(4):424–32. PubMed PMID: 21272168. Epub 2011/01/29. eng.
97. Steiner UC, Trueb RM, Schad K, Kamarashev J, Koch S, French LE, et al. Trichophyton rubrum-induced Majocchi's Granuloma in a heart transplant recipient. A therapeutic challenge. J Dermatol Case Rep. 2012;6(3):70–2. PubMed PMID: 23091582. Pubmed Central PMCID: PMC3470792. Epub 2012/10/24. eng.
98. Salim A, Reece SM, Smith AG, Harrison D, Ramsay HM, Harden PN, et al. Sebaceous hyperplasia and skin cancer in patients undergoing renal transplant. J Am Acad Dermatol. 2006;55(5):878–81. PubMed PMID: 17052497. Epub 2006/10/21. eng.
99. Hwang S, Schwartz RA. Keratosis pilaris: a common follicular hyperkeratosis. Cutis. 2008;82(3):177–80. PubMed PMID: 18856156. Epub 2008/10/17. eng.

100. Mevorah B, Marazzi A, Frenk E. The prevalence of accentuated palmoplantar markings and keratosis pilaris in atopic dermatitis, autosomal dominant ichthyosis and control dermatological patients. Br J Dermatol. 1985;112(6):679–85. PubMed PMID: 4005167. Epub 1985/06/01. eng.
101. Lally A, Casabonne D, Newton R, Wojnarowska F. Seborrheic dermatitis among Oxford renal transplant recipients. J Eur Acad Dermatol Venereol. 2010;24(5):561–4. PubMed PMID: 19888944. Epub 2009/11/06. eng.
102. Gupta AK, Bluhm R. Seborrheic dermatitis. J Eur Acad Dermatol Venereol. 2004;18(1):13–26; quiz 19–20. PubMed PMID: 14678527. Epub 2003/12/18. eng.
103. Plewig G, Jansen T. Seborrheic dermatitis. In: Wolff K, Goldsmith L, Katz SI, Gilchrest BA, Paller AS, Leffell DJ, editors. Fitzpatrick's dermatology in general medicine. 7th ed. New York: McGraw Hill Medical; 2008. p. 219–25.
104. Schaub NA, Drewe J, Sponagel L, Gilli L, Courvoisier S, Gyr N, et al. Is there a relation between risk groups or initial CD4 T cell counts and prevalence of seborrheic dermatitis in HIV-infected patients? Dermatology. 1999;198(2):126–9. PubMed PMID: 10325457. Epub 1999/05/15. eng.
105. Groisser D, Bottone EJ, Lebwohl M. Association of Pityrosporum orbiculare (Malassezia furfur) with seborrheic dermatitis in patients with acquired immunodeficiency syndrome (AIDS). J Am Acad Dermatol. 1989;20(5 Pt 1):770–3. PubMed PMID: 2523907. Epub 1989/05/01. eng.
106. Smith KJ, Skelton HG, Yeager J, Ledsky R, McCarthy W, Baxter D, et al. Cutaneous findings in HIV-1-positive patients: a 42-month prospective study. Military Medical Consortium for the Advancement of Retroviral Research (MMCARR). J Am Acad Dermatol. 1994;31(5 Pt 1):746–54. PubMed PMID: 7929920. Epub 1994/11/01. eng.
107. Guillaume JC, Karneff MC, Revuz J. Seborrheic dermatitis and cancer of the upper respiratory and digestive tracts. Ann Dermatol Venereol. 1991;118(9):607–9. PubMed PMID: 1836940. Epub 1991/01/01. Dermite seborrheique et cancers des voies aero-digestives superieures. fre.
108. Tegner E. Seborrhoeic dermatitis of the face induced by PUVA treatment. Acta Derm Venereol. 1983;63(4):335–9. PubMed PMID: 6195866. Epub 1983/01/01. eng.
109. Moehrle M, Dennenmoser B, Schlagenhauff B, Thomma S, Garbe C. High prevalence of seborrhoeic dermatitis on the face and scalp in mountain guides. Dermatology. 2000;201(2):146–7. PubMed PMID: 11053918. Epub 2000/10/29. eng.
110. Reed RJ, Leone P. Porokeratosis–a mutant clonal keratosis of the epidermis. I. Histogenesis. Arch Dermatol. 1970;101(3):340–7.
111. Stoff B, Salisbury C, Parker D, O'Reilly Zwald F. Dermatopathology of skin cancer in solid organ transplant recipients. Transplant Rev. 2010;24(4):172–89.
112. Herranz P, Pizarro A, De Lucas R, Robayna MG, Rubio FA, Sanz A, et al. High incidence of porokeratosis in renal transplant recipients. Br J Dermatol. 1997;136(2):176–9.
113. Bencini PL, Crosti C, Montagnino G, Sala F. Porokeratosis and immunosuppression. J Am Acad Dermatol. 1986;14(4):682–3. PubMed PMID: 3958281. Epub 1986/04/01. eng.
114. Proby CH. Catherine porokeratosis in organ transplant recipients. In: Otley CC, Thomas S, editors. Skin disease in organ transplantation. New York: Cambridge University Press; 2008. p. 119–21.
115. Manganoni AM, Facchetti F, Gavazzoni R. Involvement of epidermal Langerhans cells in porokeratosis of immunosuppressed renal transplant recipients. J Am Acad Dermatol. 1989;21(4 Pt 1):799–801. PubMed PMID: 2808797. Epub 1989/10/01. eng.
116. Chugh KS, Sharma SC, Singh V, Sakhuja V, Jha V, Gupta KL. Spectrum of dermatological lesions in renal allograft recipients in a tropical environment. Dermatology. 1994;188(2):108–12. PubMed PMID: 8136535. Epub 1994/01/01. eng.
117. Gilead L, Guberman D, Zlotogorski A, Vardy DA, Klaus SN. Immunosuppression-induced porokeratosis of Mibelli: complete regression of lesions upon cessation of immunosuppressive therapy. J Eur Acad Dermatol Venereol. 1995;5(2):170–2.
118. Zenarola P, Melillo L, Lomuto M, Carotenuto M, Gomes VE, Marzocchi W. Exacerbation of porokeratosis: a sign of immunodepression. J Am Acad Dermatol. 1993;29(6):1035–6. PubMed PMID: 8245238. Epub 1993/12/01. eng.
119. Sasson M, Krain AD. Porokeratosis and cutaneous malignancy: a review. Dermatol Surg. 1996; 22(4):339–42.
120. Lally A, Casabonne D, Waterboer T, Imko-Walczuk B, Michael KM, Pawlita M, et al. Association of seborrhoeic warts with skin cancer in renal transplant recipients. J Eur Acad Dermatol Venereol. 2010;24(3):302–7. PubMed PMID: 19732252. Epub 2009/09/08. eng.
121. Thyssen JP, Zachariae C. Successful treatment of multiple seborrheic keratoses using acitretin. J Eur Acad Dermatol Venereol. 2007;21(2):269–70. PubMed PMID: 17243977. Epub 2007/01/25. eng.
122. Zaenglein AL, Graber EM, Thiboutot DM, Strauss JS. Acne vulgaris and acneiform eruptions. In: Wolff KGL, Katz SI, Gilchrest BA, Paller AS, Leffell DJ, editors. Fitzpatrick's dermatology in general medicine. 7th ed. New York: McGraw Hill Publishing; 2008. p. 690–703.
123. Dessinioti C, Antoniou C, Katsambas A. Acneiform eruptions. Clin Dermatol. 2014;32(1):24–34. PubMed PMID: 24314375. Epub 2013/12/10. eng.
124. Al-Himdani S, Ud-Din S, Gilmore S, Bayat A. Striae distensae: a comprehensive review and evidence-based evaluation of prophylaxis and treatment. Br J Dermatol. 2013;11. PubMed PMID: 24125059. Epub 2013/10/16. Eng.
125. McDaniel DH, Ash K, Zukowski M. Treatment of stretch marks with the 585-nm flashlamp-pumped

pulsed dye laser. Dermatol Surg. 1996;22(4):332–7.

126. Kang S, Kim KJ, Griffiths CE, Wong TY, Talwar HS, Fisher GJ, et al. Topical tretinoin (retinoic acid) improves early stretch marks. Arch Dermatol. 1996;132(5):519–26. PubMed PMID: 8624148. Epub 1996/05/01. eng.
127. Boudou P, Fiet J, Vexiau P, Villette JM, Hardy N, Dreux C. Greater conversion of testosterone to 5 alpha-dihydrotestosterone, reflecting increased peripheral 5 alpha-reductase activity in nude mice treated with high doses of cyclosporine A. J Steroid Biochem. 1990;36(6):597–601. PubMed PMID: 2214776. Epub 1990/08/28. eng.
128. Vexiau P, Fiet J, Boudou P, Villette JM, Feutren G, Hardy N, et al. Increase in plasma 5 alpha-androstane-3 alpha,17 beta-diol glucuronide as a marker of peripheral androgen action in hirsutism: a side-effect induced by cyclosporine A. J Steroid Biochem. 1990;35(1):133–7. PubMed PMID: 2137888. Epub 1990/01/01. eng.
129. Heaphy Jr MR, Shamma HN, Hickmann M, White MJ. Cyclosporine-induced folliculodystrophy. J Am Acad Dermatol. 2004;50(2):310–5. PubMed PMID: 14726894. Epub 2004/01/17. eng.
130. Boschnakow A, May T, Assaf C, Tebbe B, Zouboulis CC. Ciclosporin A-induced sebaceous gland hyperplasia. Br J Dermatol. 2003;149(1):198–200. PubMed PMID: 12890221. Epub 2003/08/02. eng.
131. Engel F, Ellero B, Woehl-Jaegle ML, Cribier B. Diffuse sebaceous hyperplasia of the face induced by cyclosporine. Ann Dermatol Venereol. 2005;132(4):342–5. PubMed PMID: 15886561. Epub 2005/05/12. Hyperplasies sebacees profuses du visage induites par la ciclosporine. fre.
132. Bencini PL, Montagnino G, Sala F, De Vecchi A, Crosti C, Tarantino A. Cutaneous lesions in 67 cyclosporin-treated renal transplant recipients. Dermatologica. 1986;172(1):24–30. PubMed PMID: 2937664. Epub 1986/01/01. eng.
133. Leyral C, Beylot-Barry M, Vergier B, Begueret H, Dromer C, Doutre MS, et al. Cyclosporine-induced follicular eruption. Ann Dermatol Venereol. 2008;135(1):58–62. PubMed PMID: 18342076. Epub 2008/03/18. Toxidermie folliculaire a la ciclosporine. fre.
134. Bader RS, Scarborough DA. Surgical pearl: intralesional electrodesiccation of sebaceous hyperplasia. J Am Acad Dermatol. 2000;1, Part 1:127–8.
135. Alster TS, Tanzi EL. Photodynamic therapy with topical aminolevulinic acid and pulsed dye laser irradiation for sebaceous hyperplasia. J Drugs Dermatol. 2003;2(5):501–4. PubMed PMID: 14558397. Epub 2003/10/16. eng.
136. Perrett CM, McGregor J, Barlow RJ, Karran P, Proby C, Harwood CA. Topical photodynamic therapy with methyl aminolevulinate to treat sebaceous hyperplasia in an organ transplant recipient. Arch Dermatol. 2006;142(6):781–2. PubMed PMID: 16785387. Epub 2006/06/21. eng.
137. Rosian R, Goslen JB, Brodell RT. The treatment of benign sebaceous hyperplasia with the topical application of bichloracetic acid. J Dermatol Surg Oncol. 1991;17(11):876–9. PubMed PMID: 1757649. Epub 1991/11/01. eng.
138. McDonald SK, Goh MS, Chong AH. Successful treatment of cyclosporine-induced sebaceous hyperplasia with oral isotretinoin in two renal transplant recipients. Australas J Dermatol. 2011;52(3):227–30. PubMed PMID: 21834824. Epub 2011/08/13. eng.
139. Yu C, Shahsavari M, Stevens G, Liskanich R, Horowitz D. Isotretinoin as monotherapy for sebaceous hyperplasia. J Drugs Dermatol. 2010;9(6):699–701. PubMed PMID: 20645535. Epub 2010/07/22. eng.
140. Lally A, Wojnarowska F. Hypertrophic pseudofolliculitis in white renal transplant recipients. Clin Exp Dermatol. 2007;32(3):268–71. PubMed PMID: 17355278. Epub 2007/03/16. eng.
141. Chua S, Affleck A, Kulkarni K. Florid hyperplastic folliculitis on the chin in a male renal transplant patient. Clin Exp Dermatol. 2008;33(1):98–9. PubMed PMID: 18039343. Epub 2007/11/28. eng.
142. Chastain MA, Millikan LE. Pilomatrix dysplasia in an immunosuppressed patient. J Am Acad Dermatol. 2000;43(1 Pt 1):118–22. PubMed PMID: 10863236. Epub 2000/06/23. eng.
143. Voulgari PV, Drosos AA. Gingival hyperplasia associated with cyclosporin A. J Rheumatol. 2002;29(11):2466. PubMed PMID: 12415611. Epub 2002/11/05. eng.
144. Kwun WH, Suh BY, Kwun KB. Effect of azithromycin in the treatment of cyclosporine-induced gingival hyperplasia in renal transplant recipients. Transplant Proc. 2003;35(1):311–2. PubMed PMID: 12591416. Epub 2003/02/20. eng.
145. Tokgoz B, Sari HI, Yildiz O, Aslan S, Sipahioglu M, Okten T, et al. Effects of azithromycin on cyclosporine-induced gingival hyperplasia in renal transplant patients. Transplant Proc. 2004;36(9):2699–702. PubMed PMID: 15621128. Epub 2004/12/29. eng.
146. Tricot L, Lebbe C, Pillebout E, Martinez F, Legendre C, Thervet E. Tacrolimus-induced alopecia in female kidney-pancreas transplant recipients. Transplantation. 2005;80(11):1546–9. PubMed PMID: 16371923. Epub 2005/12/24. eng.
147. Ushigome H, Yoshimura N, Okamoto M, Najima H, Hamajima T, Nakai I, et al. Two cases of tacrolimus-induced alopecia following kidney transplantation. Transplant Proc. 1999;31(7):2885–6. PubMed PMID: 10578326. Epub 1999/12/01. eng.
148. Talbot D, Rix D, Abusin K, Mirza D, Manas D. Alopecia as a consequence of tacrolimus therapy in renal transplantation? Transplantation. 1997;64(11):1631–2. PubMed PMID: 9415574. Epub 1998/02/12. eng.
149. Bumbacea RS, Ghiordanescu I. Atopic dermatitis induced by systemic immunosuppression with tacrolimus – case report. Eur Ann Allergy Clin Immunol. 2013;45(3):109–10. PubMed PMID: 23862401. Epub 2013/07/19. eng.
150. Ponte GM, Baidal DA, Romanelli P, Faradji RN, Poggioli R, Cure P, et al. Resolution of severe atopic dermatitis after tacrolimus withdrawal. Cell

Transplant. 2007;16(1):23–30. PubMed PMID: 17436852. Epub 2007/04/18. eng.
151. Ahn IS, Chung BY, Cho SI, Kim HO, Park CW, Lee CH. Epidermal cysts in a tacrolimus treated renal transplant recipient. Ann Dermatol. 2011;23 Suppl 2:S182–4. PubMed PMID: 22148045. Pubmed Central PMCID: PMC3229060. Epub 2011/12/08. eng.
152. Campistol JM, de Fijter JW, Flechner SM, Langone A, Morelon E, Stockfleth E. mTOR inhibitor-associated dermatologic and mucosal problems. Clin Transplant. 2010;24(2):149–56. PubMed PMID: 20236129. Epub 2010/03/20. eng.
153. Mahe E, Morelon E, Lechaton S, Kreis H, De Prost Y, Bodemer C. Sirolimus-induced onychopathy in renal transplant recipients. Ann Dermatol Venereol. 2006;133(6–7):531–5. PubMed PMID: 16885839. Epub 2006/08/04. Onychopathie associee au sirolimus chez les transplantes renaux. fre.
154. Euvrard S, Morelon E, Rostaing L, Goffin E, Brocard A, Tromme I, et al. Sirolimus and secondary skin-cancer prevention in kidney transplantation. N Engl J Med. 2012;367(4):329–39. PubMed PMID: 22830463. Epub 2012/07/27. eng.
155. Schaffellner S, Jakoby E, Kniepeiss D, Stadlbauer V, Duller D, Iberer F, et al. Center experience in liver transplantation (LTX): management of dermal side effects caused by sirolimus. Int Immunopharmacol. 2005;5(1):137–40. PubMed PMID: 15589473. Epub 2004/12/14. eng.
156. Mahe E, Morelon E, Lechaton S, Drappier JC, de Prost Y, Kreis H, et al. Acne in recipients of renal transplantation treated with sirolimus: clinical, microbiologic, histologic, therapeutic, and pathogenic aspects. J Am Acad Dermatol. 2006;55(1):139–42. PubMed PMID: 16781309. Epub 2006/06/20. eng.
157. Mahe E, Morelon E, Lechaton S, Sang KH, Mansouri R, Ducasse MF, et al. Cutaneous adverse events in renal transplant recipients receiving sirolimus-based therapy. Transplantation. 2005;79(4):476–82. PubMed PMID: 15729175. Epub 2005/02/25. eng.
158. Kunzle N, Venetz JP, Pascual M, Panizzon RG, Laffitte E. Sirolimus-induced acneiform eruption. Dermatology. 2005;211(4):366–9. PubMed PMID: 16286750. Epub 2005/11/16. eng.
159. Nomura M, He Z, Koyama I, Ma WY, Miyamoto K, Dong Z. Involvement of the Akt/mTOR pathway on EGF-induced cell transformation. Mol Carcinog. 2003;38(1):25–32. PubMed PMID: 12949840. Epub 2003/09/02. eng.
160. Hardinger KL, Cornelius LA, Trulock 3rd EP, Brennan DC. Sirolimus-induced leukocytoclastic vasculitis. Transplantation. 2002;74(5):739–43. PubMed PMID: 12352895. Epub 2002/09/28. eng.
161. Pasqualotto AC, Bianco PD, Sukiennik TC, Furian R, Garcia VD. Sirolimus-induced leukocytoclastic vasculitis: the second case reported. Am J Transplant. 2004;4(9):1549–51. PubMed PMID: 15307846. Epub 2004/08/17. eng.
162. Euvrard S, Boissonnat P, Roussoulieres A, Kanitakis J, Decullier E, Claudy A, et al. Effect of everolimus on skin cancers in calcineurin inhibitor-treated heart transplant recipients. Transpl Int. 2010;23(8):855–7. PubMed PMID: 19951373. Epub 2009/12/03. eng.
163. Yee KW, Hymes SR, Heller L, Prieto VG, Welch MA, Giles FJ. Cutaneous leukocytoclastic vasculitis in a patient with myelodysplastic syndrome after therapy with the rapamycin analogue everolimus: case report and review of the literature. Leuk Lymphoma. 2006;47(5):926–9. PubMed PMID: 16753882. Epub 2006/06/07. eng.
164. Imuran (azathioprine) [package insert]. San Diego: Prometheus Laboratories Inc.; 2011.
165. Lawson DH, Lovatt GE, Gurton CS, Hennings RC. Adverse effects of azathioprine. Adverse Drug React Acute Poisoning Rev. 1984;3(3):161–71. PubMed PMID: 6397980. Epub 1984/01/01. eng.
166. de Fonclare AL, Khosrotehrani K, Aractingi S, Duriez P, Cosnes J, Beaugerie L. Erythema nodosum-like eruption as a manifestation of azathioprine hypersensitivity in patients with inflammatory bowel disease. Arch Dermatol. 2007;143(6):744–8. PubMed PMID: 17576940. Epub 2007/06/20. eng.
167. van Gelder T, ter Meulen CG, Hene R, Weimar W, Hoitsma A. Oral ulcers in kidney transplant recipients treated with sirolimus and mycophenolate mofetil. Transplantation. 2003;75(6):788–91. PubMed PMID: 12660502. Epub 2003/03/28. eng.
168. Rault R. Mycophenolate-associated onycholysis. Ann Intern Med. 2000;133(11):921–2. PubMed PMID: 11103069. Epub 2000/12/05. eng.
169. Semhoun-Ducloux S, Ducloux D, Miguet JP. Mycophenolate mofetil-induced dyshidrotic eczema. Ann Intern Med. 2000;132(5):417. PubMed PMID: 10691595. Epub 2000/02/26. eng.
170. Desai A, Kartono F, Del Rosso JQ. Systemic retinoid therapy: a status report on optimal use and safety of long-term therapy. Dermatol Clin. 2007;25(2):185–93, vi. PubMed PMID: 17430755. Epub 2007/04/14. eng.
171. George R, Weightman W, Russ GR, Bannister KM, Mathew TH. Acitretin for chemoprevention of non-melanoma skin cancers in renal transplant recipients. Australas J Dermatol. 2002;43(4):269–73. PubMed PMID: 12423433. Epub 2002/11/09. eng.
172. McKenna DB, Murphy GM. Skin cancer chemoprophylaxis in renal transplant recipients: 5 years of experience using low-dose acitretin. Br J Dermatol. 1999;140(4):656–60. PubMed PMID: 10233316. Epub 1999/05/08. eng.
173. Marquez C, Bair SM, Smithberger E, Cherpelis BS, Glass LF. Systemic retinoids for chemoprevention of non-melanoma skin cancer in high-risk patients. J Drugs Dermatol. 2010;9(7):753–8. PubMed PMID: 20677528. Epub 2010/08/04. eng.
174. Goulden V, Layton AM, Cunliffe WJ. Long-term safety of isotretinoin as a treatment for acne vulgaris. Br J Dermatol. 1994;131(3):360–3. PubMed PMID: 7918010. Epub 1994/09/01. eng.
175. Otley CC, Stasko T, Tope WD, Lebwohl M. Chemoprevention of nonmelanoma skin cancer with systemic retinoids: practical dosing and management of adverse effects. Dermatol Surg.

2006;32(4):562–8. PubMed PMID: 16681667. Epub 2006/05/10. eng.
176. Epaulard O, Leccia MT, Blanche S, Chosidow O, Mamzer-Bruneel MF, Ravaud P, et al. Phototoxicity and photocarcinogenesis associated with voriconazole. Med Mal Infect. 2011;41(12):639–45. PubMed PMID: 22055586. Epub 2011/11/08. eng.
177. Lankerani L, Baron ED. Photosensitivity to exogenous agents. J Cutan Med Surg. 2004;8(6):424–31. PubMed PMID: 15988550. Epub 2005/07/01. eng.
178. Epaulard O, Saint-Raymond C, Villier C, Charles J, Roch N, Beani JC, et al. Multiple aggressive squamous cell carcinomas associated with prolonged voriconazole therapy in four immunocompromised patients. Clin Microbiol Infect. 2010;16(9):1362–4. PubMed PMID: 19930272. Epub 2009/11/26. eng.
179. Scholz I, Oberwittler H, Riedel KD, Burhenne J, Weiss J, Haefeli WE, et al. Pharmacokinetics, metabolism and bioavailability of the triazole antifungal agent voriconazole in relation to CYP2C19 genotype. Br J Clin Pharmacol. 2009;68(6):906–15. PubMed PMID: 20002085. Pubmed Central PMCID: PMC2810802. Epub 2009/12/17. eng.
180. Ibrahim SF, Singer JP, Arron ST. Catastrophic squamous cell carcinoma in lung transplant patients treated with voriconazole. Dermatol Surg. 2010;36(11):1752–5. PubMed PMID: 20533939. Pubmed Central PMCID: PMC3046628. Epub 2010/06/11. eng.
181. Miller DD, Cowen EW, Nguyen JC, McCalmont TH, Fox LP. Melanoma associated with long-term voriconazole therapy: a new manifestation of chronic photosensitivity. Arch Dermatol. 2010;146(3):300–4. PubMed PMID: 20083676. Epub 2010/01/20. eng.
182. Morice C, Acher A, Soufir N, Michel M, Comoz F, Leroy D, et al. Multifocal aggressive squamous cell carcinomas induced by prolonged voriconazole therapy: a case report. Case Rep Med. 2010;2010:351084. PubMed PMID: 21209800. Pubmed Central PMCID: PMC3014742. Epub 2011/01/07. eng.
183. Feist A, Lee R, Osborne S, Lane J, Yung G. Increased incidence of cutaneous squamous cell carcinoma in lung transplant recipients taking long-term voriconazole. J Heart Lung Transplant. 2012;31(11):1177–81. PubMed PMID: 22841559. Epub 2012/07/31. eng.
184. Zwald FO, Brown M. Skin cancer in solid organ transplant recipients: advances in therapy and management: part II. Management of skin cancer in solid organ transplant recipients. J Am Acad Dermatol. 2011;65(2):263–79; quiz 80. PubMed PMID: 21763562. Epub 2011/07/19. eng.
185. Muehleisen B, Pazhenkottil A, French LE, Hofbauer GF. Nonmelanoma skin cancer in organ transplant recipients: increase without delay after transplant and subsequent acceleration. JAMA Dermatol. 2013;149(5):618–20. PubMed PMID: 23677099. Epub 2013/05/17. eng.
186. Park GH, Chang SE, Won CH, Lee MW, Choi JH, Moon KC, et al. Incidence of primary skin cancer after organ transplantation: an 18-year single-center experience in Korea. J Am Acad Dermatol. 2013;13. PubMed PMID: 24342756. Epub 2013/12/18. Eng.
187. Piselli P, Busnach G, Fratino L, Citterio F, Ettorre GM, De Paoli P, et al. De novo malignancies after organ transplantation: focus on viral infections. Curr Mol Med. 2013;13(7):1217–27. PubMed PMID: 23278452. Epub 2013/01/03. eng.
188. Engelhardt C, Curiel-Lewandrowski C, Warneke J, Cranmer L. Metastatic cutaneous squamous cell carcinoma responding to erlotinib therapy. J Am Acad Dermatol. 2011;65(1):237–8. PubMed PMID: 21679836. Epub 2011/06/18. eng.
189. Dorsey K, Agulnik M. Promising new molecular targeted therapies in head and neck cancer. Drugs. 2013;73(4):315–25. PubMed PMID: 23440867. Epub 2013/02/27. eng.
190. Shaib W, Kono S, Saba N. Antiepidermal growth factor receptor therapy in squamous cell carcinoma of the head and neck. J Oncol. 2012;2012:521215. PubMed PMID: 22778735. Pubmed Central PMCID: PMC3388373. Epub 2012/07/11. eng.
191. Hu JC, Sadeghi P, Pinter-Brown LC, Yashar S, Chiu MW. Cutaneous side effects of epidermal growth factor receptor inhibitors: clinical presentation, pathogenesis, and management. J Am Acad Dermatol. 2007;56(2):317–26. PubMed PMID: 17141360. Epub 2006/12/05. eng.
192. Curry JL, Torres-Cabala CA, Kim KB, Tetzlaff MT, Duvic M, Tsai KY, et al. Dermatologic toxicities to targeted cancer therapy: shared clinical and histologic adverse skin reactions. Int J Dermatol. 2013;24. PubMed PMID: 23879247. Epub 2013/07/25. Eng.
193. Potthoff K, Hofheinz R, Hassel JC, Volkenandt M, Lordick F, Hartmann JT, et al. Interdisciplinary management of EGFR-inhibitor-induced skin reactions: a German expert opinion. Ann Oncol. 2011;22(3):524–35. PubMed PMID: 20709812. Epub 2010/08/17. eng.
194. Tomkova H, Kohoutek M, Zabojnikova M, Pospiskova M, Ostrizkova L, Gharibyar M. Cetuximab-induced cutaneous toxicity. J Eur Acad Dermatol Venereol. 2010;24(6):692–6. PubMed PMID: 19925598. Epub 2009/11/21. eng.
195. Scope A, Agero AL, Dusza SW, Myskowski PL, Lieb JA, Saltz L, et al. Randomized double-blind trial of prophylactic oral minocycline and topical tazarotene for cetuximab-associated acne-like eruption. J Clin Oncol. 2007;25(34):5390–6. PubMed PMID: 18048820. Epub 2007/12/01. eng.

Advances in Photoprotection

2

Gillian M. Murphy and Oonagh Molloy

Contents

G.M. Murphy, MD, FRCPI, FRCP, Edin (✉)
O. Molloy, MB, MICGP
National Photobiology Unit, Department of Dermatology, Beaumont and Mater Misericordiae Hospital, Dublin, Ireland
e-mail: gillianmmurphy@gmail.com; molloyoona@yahoo.co.uk

2.1 Introduction

Malignant melanoma and non-melanoma skin cancer rates have increased in Caucasian populations worldwide, with an exaggerated increase in those living in lower-latitude climates. In recent times, global awareness of this growing epidemic has gathered prominence. Many countries have introduced UVR occupational safety legislation (EU). Furthermore, legal requirements for UV standard glass, UV protective eyewear and legislating for the regulation of indoor tanning may reduce UVR exposure. Educating populations on the hazards of UVR exposure has been shown to be effective. Most European countries, Australia and the United States campaign annually to remind the public of the need to reduce exposure.

Other causes of skin cancer are listed in Table 2.1.

2.2 Ultraviolet Radiation and Carcinogenesis

UVR is a complete carcinogen, with the ability to initiate, promote and lead to progression of a skin cancer independent of other risk factors [2, 3].

The ultraviolet spectrum encompasses UVC (200–280 nm), UVB (280–315 nm) and UVA (315–400 nm). UVC is absorbed by stratospheric ozone except in areas with ozone depletion such as the Antarctic. UVB is the predominant cause of skin cancer but UVA is increasingly implicated

F. Zwald, M.D. Brown (eds.), *Advances in Transplant Dermatology: Clinical and Practical Implications*, DOI 10.1007/978-3-319-12445-2_2, © Springer International Publishing Switzerland 2015

Table 2.1 Genetic predisposition to skin cancer development, e.g. Gorlin's syndrome (basal cell naevus syndrome), xeroderma pigmentosum

Immunosuppression
Hydrocarbons (industrial tar)
Ionising radiation
Arsenic (contained in the tonic 'Parish's food', available until the 1960s)
Smoking
Chronic ulceration
Oncogenic HPV
Human herpesvirus 8 (HHV-8) responsible for Kaposi's sarcoma
PUVA (psoralen + UVA) used in the treatment of psoriasis

because of the ability of UVA to penetrate deeply into the dermis and the sheer amount of UVA, one hundred-fold greater than UVB [4], to which people are exposed. UVA has been implicated in photoaging [5] but is seen to have an overlapping effect with UVB, leading to a summative carcinogenic effect.

2.3 Mutations

The initial event in photo-carcinogenesis occurs when UVR of a specific wavelength is absorbed by epidermal cellular deoxyribonucleic acid (DNA), causing the formation of cyclobutane pyrimidine dimers (CPDs) in the DNA double helix [6]. Ineffective removal of these CPDs can lead to errors in DNA transcription. DNA replication and repair is a complex process of enzyme-dependant pathways, which prevent abnormal DNA synthesis by nucleotide excision repair (NER) [7]. The process of NER and excised pyrimidine dimers (PDs) is shown to be immuno-protective [8]. Under normal conditions during replication, DNA is unzipped, the thymine dimer repaired, and DNA is then reconstituted hopefully without error, but the repair mechanism is error prone and may be overwhelmed by UVR damage. Aging skin also does not repair itself as readily and is less efficient at removing harmful CPDs than younger skin [9]. UVR-induced mutations in gene sequences lead to tumour suppressor proteins including p53, changing from protective genes into oncogenes. Mutated DNA ultimately leads to skin cancers.

2.4 Apoptosis

The body's second mechanism of defence against abnormal or cancerous cells is the activation of the intrinsic apoptotic pathway, whereby cells beyond repair are eliminated by a non-inflammatory mechanism in contrast to necrosis which is an inflammatory process [10]. Apoptosis is triggered via p53 protein to prevent further abnormal DNA replication.

It is mediated by the caspase protease cascade, with protein p53 causing cell cycle arrest in S1 by producing p21.

2.5 Immunosuppression

The immunosuppressive effects of UVR were elegantly demonstrated by Margaret Kripke. Syngeneic mice were either UVB irradiated or non-irradiated. Skin cancer transplants were carried out in both groups. The non-irradiated group rejected the tumour, whereas the UVR-irradiated group failed to reject the transplanted skin tumour [11]. This inability to recognise skin cancer as a foreign antigen was demonstrated to be transferable by lymphocytes [12], suggesting that, in squamous cell carcinoma (SCC), this is an antigenic process and possibly explains why SCC is disproportionately represented in organ transplant recipients (OTRs), who are immunosuppressed to prevent rejection of the graft.

Langerhans cells, a specific type of dendritic cell within the epidermis, act as antigen-presenting cells and have an integral role in local immune surveillance. UVR is known to deplete Langerhans cell populations within the epidermis [13]. Failure of this normal effect, with Langerhans cell resistance to UVR, leads to development of polymorphic light eruption (PLE) [14]. It is thought that this genetic aberration may have a protective effect against the development of skin cancer [15].

Urocanic acid, found in its *trans-isomer* in the skin, when exposed to UVB (action spectrum), changes to its *cis-isomer*, which is highly immunosuppressive and may suppress contact hypersensitivity and delayed hypersensitivity through TNF-a [16, 17]. UVR may modulate growth factors and cytokines such as TNF-a and interleukins (ILs), especially IL-10, and activate receptors for Fas, TNF-a, IL-1 and the melanocortin receptor, which regulates pigment in the skin.

Both UVB and UVA are immunosuppressive and abrogate cell-mediated responses. Consequently, human papilloma virus (HPV) is augmented on immunosuppressed skin. Indeed, the interaction of UVR immunosuppression with high-risk human papilloma virus (HPV) subtypes may induce skin cancers on keratinized squamous epithelium [18]. Warts are more common in the immunosuppressed, being particularly associated with azathioprine. HPV has the ability to block the BAK signalling pathway, which represents a key cellular defence in activating the apoptotic pathway, thereby rendering it prone to facilitating carcinogenesis [19]. In addition, it also effects programmed cell death, allowing old cells to survive when they normally would not [20].

2.6 Organ Transplant Recipients

OTRs have between a 65-fold and 250-fold increased risk of SCC [21, 22].

This is the inverse of the natural order of occurrence in skin cancer subtypes, with basal cell carcinomas (BCCs) occurring at 3-fold the rate of SCCs, within an immunocompetent population. The OTR group is at particular increased risk of skin cancer because of the reduction of immune surveillance by immunosuppressive drugs. Immunosuppression coupled with UVR – which has local and systemic immunosuppressive effects – augments cancer risk.

2.7 Sun Exposure Patterns

Intentional sun exposure is the deliberate attempt of an individual to be exposed to the sun usually with the express desire to acquire a tan. The difficulty in relation to tanning is that the dose required to tan is close to the same dose known to cause sunburn. The action spectrum of erythema is similar to the absorption spectrum of DNA and DNA is the chromophore for sunburn [6]. Both burning and tanning are caused by thymine dimer formation. It is impossible, therefore, to tan without causing DNA damage, thus promoting the development of skin cancer. The World Health Organization and public health campaigns have been actively engaged in initiatives to reduce direct and inadvertent UVR exposure, such as sunsmart.com or the 'slip, slop, slap' campaign – slip on a shirt, slop on sunscreen, slap on a hat. Sunbathing first gained popularity in the late nineteenth century as a medical treatment to prevent vitamin D–dependant rickets and during recovery from tuberculosis. Finsen first used artificial UV lamps for this purpose for which he received the Nobel Prize [23].

Sunbathing and the desire to be tanned began to be affiliated with affluence and a sense of well-being. Indeed, Coco Chanel is credited with making a tan fashionable in the 1900s, which has persisted to this day. Prior to this, tanned skin was associated with outdoor labour and lower social standing. From a social standpoint, attitudinal surveys towards tanning in Ireland have revealed perceptions that a tanned appearance makes one appear thinner and more attractive [24]. This is likely to have influenced the trend for indoor tanning which is achieved by exposure to predominantly UVA light.

There have been major concerns in relation to sunbed use and melanoma risk especially in those aged under 35 [25].

To date, the use of indoor tanning has largely gone unregulated until recently. Some countries have introduced legislation to regulate and in some instances outlaw its use. In Ireland, the Public Health (Sunbeds) Act 2014 has been enacted into legislation by the Dail (Irish House of Representatives) and the Seanad (the Irish Senate) with effect from the 21st of July, 2014 [1]. This Act aims to regulate the use and supply of sunbeds and outlaws the use of sunbeds in persons under the age of 18 years [26]. In Australia a measure is being sought to outlaw indoor tanning practices completely, because of the high burden of disease

Table 2.2 Factors influencing UVR intensity

Time of day
Latitude
Altitude
Season
Cloud cover
Air pollution
Transmission of UVR through glass and water
Rayleigh scattering (gives the daytime sky its blue colour)
Ozone depletion

and morbidity among the fair-skinned population. Reduction of UVR may be achieved by an understanding of the factors influencing UVR dose. Factors influencing UVR intensity are listed in Table 2.2.

Unintentional UV exposure occurs with outdoor occupation, recreation and exercise and is often disregarded by the individual. The cumulative dose can be significant over decades and particularly relevant with lifestyle after retirement, which may have a large outdoor component [27, 28]. There appears to be a latent period between high sun exposure and the development of skin cancer of between 10 and 15 years [29].

Countries such as Australia, where a large fair-skinned population have been shown to have significantly higher rates of non-melanoma skin cancers and melanoma, have had success in reducing intentional and unintentional sun exposure, whereas countries with intermittently high UVR levels have a greater problem.

Individuals may be quite unaware of the potential risks of unintentional sun exposure and do not take the necessary precautions. It is worth noting that the outdoor occupational exposure risk amounts to four times that of the indoor worker. A recent paper looking at occupational UVR exposure patterns in Irish and Danish gardeners demonstrated lower UVR exposure in the Irish group, probably due to indoor breaks at peak UVR hours, compared to their Danish counterparts [30]. Scheduling outdoor work to coincide with trough UV hours is an important occupational health consideration.

Table 2.3 Strategies for sun avoidance

Avoid sun at peak UV hours between 11 a.m. and 3 p.m.
Seek shade when one's shadow is shorter than one's height
Wear protective clothing, hats and eyewear in peak sunlight hours
Apply sunscreen regularly and liberally to sun-exposed areas

The development of the Global UV index provides daily geographic information on UV intensity in any particular location [31]. This serves as a guide to high-risk exposure times. Drawing attention to unintentional sun exposure and explaining its damaging effects may lead to modification of exposure and very significant reductions in lifetime dose.

2.8 Strategies for Sun Avoidance (Table 2.3)

2.8.1 Clothing

Exercise and outdoor activities are good for individual health.

The style of garment influences the area of skin exposed. Ideal garments for peak sun times are high necked, long sleeved and full length. Fabrics vary widely. See-through and open-weave fabrics transmit UVR. The ultraviolet protection factor (UPF) is the ratio of the intensity of UVR before and after passing through a fabric and is principally determined by the size of aperture in the weave [32, 33]. A crude measurement of UPF may be ascertained by holding a material up to direct sunlight and assessing the amount of light that penetrates through it. Simply, the tighter the weave, the higher its protectiveness. For example, denim is a very effective barrier against UVR penetration but may be poorly tolerated in hot climates. In contrast some cotton T-shirts may actually transmit UVR especially when wet. As an alternative, the UPF of a fabric may be enhanced artificially by incorporating sunscreen particles, such as titanium dioxide (TiO_2), onto fibres. Some fabrics now carry a

Table 2.4 Sequelae of ultraviolet light on eye structures

Cataracts
Photokeratitis
Pterygium
Solar retinopathy
Pingueculae

UPF rating, although UVA rating is more difficult to quantify. International recommendations for a sun-protective fabric suggest a UPF of >40 and a desired reduction of UVA exposure to ~5 %.

2.8.2 Sunglasses

Sun-protective eyewear with UV protective lenses are important in reducing the deleterious effect of UV light to the delicate structures of the eye [34], as shown in Table 2.4. It is estimated that the number of cataracts could be reduced by prudent use of UV protective eyewear [35].

Adequate eyecover with sunglasses requires a wide side handle to protect the lateral aspect of the eye from photodamage, in addition to UV protective lenses. The recommendation is a lens which absorbs up to 400 nm of UVR. Large-sized lenses and wrap-around designs are better. Sunglasses should come with a standardised UV rating, bearing a safety mark, e.g. CE, for European products or an international equivalent.

The same should apply to snow goggles.

2.8.3 Hats

Hats have been worn throughout history, particularly up until the turn of the twentieth century. They are rarely worn now in the western world, with significant consequences for those chronically exposed sites, such as scalp, neck and face. Scientific studies looking at the wearing of hats have clearly demonstrated a benefit in reduction of the development of skin cancer, in high-risk sites, if a broad-brimmed hat (at least 7 cm) is worn [36].

Caps fail to protect the sides of the face, ears and neck.

2.8.4 Sunscreens

There has been much debate about the real therapeutic benefit of sunscreen use. The ideal sunscreen should protect against UVA and UVB, should deliver what it sets out to achieve, should be acceptable to its target to enhance compliance and should adhere to standards and safety requirements. The minimal erythema dose (MED) is the amount of UVR required to induce barely perceptible erythema on exposed skin [37]. The sun protection factor (SPF) refers to the ratio of the minimal erythema dose (MED) of solar radiation on skin treated with sunscreen divided by the MED on untreated skin. It is important to state that the SPF/UVB relationship is not linear – a common public misconception – with ineffective application of sunscreen leading to a sub-optimal actual SPF [38, 39] (Fig. 2.1).

UVB is significantly (1,000 times) [40] more biologically active while UVA is responsible for sunburn and producing erythema, and thus SPF reflects protection for the most part from UVB [41]. The amount of sunscreen applied determines the SPF. Sunscreens are tested with 2 mg of sunscreen/cm^2 of skin [42]. If less than this is used, there is much greater penetration of UVR than one might think. Sunscreen application technique is notoriously poor in practice, with too little applied, unevenness of application and some areas totally missed being the norm [42, 43]. Education helps to minimise such errors.

Protection from UVA is more difficult to quantify. In vivo, UVA protection is measured as persistent pigment darkening. The Diffey method measures UVA protection using an in vitro test and is represented by a 5* rating. This method measures the flatness of spectral absorbance of a sunscreen across UVA and UVB and the star rating is calculated as a ratio of UVA/UVB absorbance [40, 49].

European recommendations suggest that the UVA-PF/SPF ratio should be >1/3. For example, a 5* rating has a ratio of 0.9. The critical wavelength is the wavelength at which 90 % of UVA and UVB is absorbed by a sunscreen. A sunscreen may be classified as broad spectrum if its

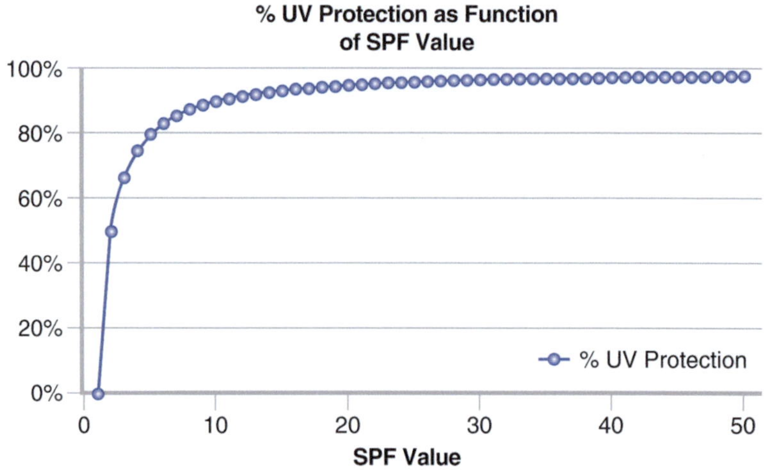

Fig. 2.1 % UV protection as function of SPF (Modified from Copyright FDA 2012)

critical wavelength measures >370 nm [38–40]. Strict labelling requirements give critical information regarding sun protection offered by a product.

Non-erythema doses of UVR are still hazardous. In fact, suberythemal doses of UVA and UVB have been shown to induce skin tumours in mice and even those with skin types IV and V and may develop skin cancers from cumulative lifetime doses of UVA.

2.8.5 Physical Sunscreens

Physical (inorganic/insoluble) sunscreens act by absorbing, reflecting and scattering UV light away from the skin. This is achieved by forming a barrier of inert mineral particles such as titanium dioxide or zinc oxide [46].

These are well tolerated and are the sunscreen of choice in those with sensitive or allergic skin types and pose less problems than the original para-aminobenzoic acid (PABA) sunscreens implicated in photoallergy.

Compliance with physical sunscreens has been an issue, as the cosmetic appearance is chalky white in colour; however, this problem has been in part overcome with novel micronized versions now available, though with the caveat that they are less protective against UVA. The addition of tinted pigments to sunscreens, for example, Dundee sunscreen, improves its appearance and its acceptability.

List of UV Filters Approved by the European Commission

Camphor benzalkonium methosulfate
Homosalate
Oxybenzone
Ensulizole
Ecamsule
Avobenzone
Benzylidene camphor sulfonic acid
Octocrilene
Polyacryloyldimethyl benzylidene camphor
Octinoxate
PEG-25 PABA
Amiloxate
Ethylhexyl triazone
Drometrizole trisiloxane
Iscotrizinol
Enzacamene
3-Benzylidene camphor
Octisalate
Padimate O
Sulisobenzone
Bisoctrizole
Bisdisulizole disodium
Bemotrizinol
Polysilicone-15
Titanium dioxide
Diethylamino hydroxybenzoyl hexyl benzoate

List of UV Filters Approved by the FDA 2012

Avobenzone
Dioxybenzone
Ecamsule

Meramidate
Oxybenzone
Sulisobenzone
Homosalate
Ensulizole
Octinoxate
Octisalate
Cinoxate
Octocrylene PABA
Padimate O
Trolamine salicylate
Ensulizole
Zinc oxide
Titanium dioxide

2.8.6 Chemical Sunscreens

Chemical (organic/soluble) sunscreen filters work by absorbing UV photons which change their electrochemical state, resulting in the emission of chemical energy in the form of heat or light. These are cosmetically more acceptable but are more likely to cause adverse reactions including allergic irritant, as well as photoallergic reactions.

Broad-spectrum sun filters are useful in preventing symptoms in photodermatoses sufferers, especially when used consistently in appropriate amounts. The difficulty remains in achieving a homogeneous coverage [42, 43]. Dihydroxyacetone (fake tan), which is usually evenly applied, provides a low SPF 2–3 [44, 45]. UVA contributes significantly to photoaging and perhaps highlighting this cosmetic aspect of UVA damage may attenuate at-risk behaviour [46]. Sunscreen on its own is not enough in reducing overall UV exposure and other strategies must be employed.

The Australian Nambour Skin Cancer Trial by Prof. Adele Green et al. revealed a lower rate of SCC development with the daily application of sunscreen, in an immunocompetent group. This was a randomised controlled trial (RCT) with originally 2,095 participants, 1,621 being followed up for an 8-year period after trial completion. It was in the extended follow-up period that a 40 % reduction in new SCC development was found in the daily sunscreen group [29]. Multiple trials, including a small RCT in Texas comprised of 50 volunteers, looked at the development of new actinic keratoses (A.Ks) in a group using daily SPF 29 or sunscreen base. A 36 % reduction in the development of new AKs was found in the intervention group [47].

2.8.7 Oral Photoprotection

The challenges of achieving homogenous sunscreen cover in topical photoprotection have spurred interest in developing oral and systemic forms of photoprotection. To date, none has translated into mainstream clinical practice. The search for a reliable oral photoprotective treatment remains ongoing.

2.8.8 Sun Avoidance

Strategies to reduce UVR exposure are quite simple.

Individuals should avoid sun at peak UV hours between 11 a.m. and 3 p.m. Adequate protective clothing, hats and eyewear are recommended in addition to seeking shade during high-intensity UVR. Applying sunscreen to sun-exposed sites in adequate amounts and at regular intervals does not provide absolute protection but rather serves as an adjunct to the above strategies [29].

Photoprotection remains a vital measure to minimise the extensive damage caused by ultraviolet light on exposed human skin [50, 51] in technology of sunscreens, and potential oral alternatives are continuing as there is a need for consistent and reliable photoprotection. Health promotion by public health, national bodies and medical doctors is vital in educating individuals on the hazards and long-term implications of UVR exposure.

References

1. Cancer in Ireland 2013: annual report of the national cancer registry. Chapter 4.1. www.ncri.ie.
2. Forbes PD, Davies RE, Urbach F. Experimental ultraviolet photocarcinogenesis: wavelength interac-

tions and time-dose relationships. Natl Cancer Inst Monogr. 1978;50:31–8.
3. El Ghissassi F, et al. A review of human carcinogens a part D: radiation. Lancet Oncol. 2009;10:751–2.
4. Poon TSC, Barnetson RSC, Halliday GM. Sunlight induced immunosuppression in humans is initially because of UVB, then UVA, followed by interactive effects. J Invest Dermatol. 2005;125:840–6.
5. Halliday GM, Rana S. Waveband and dose dependency of sunlight-induced immunomodulation and cellular changes. Photochem Photobiol. 2008;84:35–46.
6. Young AR, et al. The similarity of action spectra for thymidine dimers in human epidermis and erythema suggests that DNA is the chromophore for erythema. J Invest Dermatol. 1998;111(6):982–8.
7. Leibeling D, Laspe P, Emmett S. Nucleotide excision repair and cancer. J Mol Histol. 2006;37(5–7):225–38.
8. Yarosh D, et al. Effect of topically applied T4 endonuclease V in liposomes on skin cancer in xeroderma pigmentosum: a randomised study. Xeroderma Pigmentosum Study Group. Lancet. 2001;357(9260):926–9.
9. Yamada M, et al. Aged human skin removes UVB-induced pyrimidine dimers from the epidermis more slowly than younger adult skin in vivo. Arch Dermatol Res. 2006;297(7):294–302.
10. Melnikova VO, Ananthaswamy HN. Cellular and molecular events leading to the development of skin cancer. Mutat Res. 2005;571(1–2):91–106.
11. Fisher S, Kripke ML. Systemic alteration induced by mice by ultraviolet light irradiation and its relationship to ultraviolet carcinogenesis. Proc Natl Acad Sci U S A. 1977;74(4):1688–92.
12. Ghoreishi M, et al. Tolerance induction by transcutaneous immunisation through ultraviolet a irradiated skin is transferable through CD4+ CD25+ T regulatory cells on host derived IL-10. J Immunol. 2006;176:2635–44.
13. Murphy GM, et al. Low dose ultraviolet B irradiation depletes human epidermal langerhans cells. Br J Dermatol. 1993;129(6):674–7.
14. Vink A, Berg R, de Gruijl F. Detection of thymine dimers in suprabasal and basal cells of chronically UV-B exposed hairless mice. J Invest Dermatol. 1993;100:795–9.
15. Lembo S, et al. Polymorphic light eruption and skin cancer prevalence: is one protective against the other? Br J Dermatol. 2008;159(6):1342–7.
16. McLoone P, et al. An action spectrum for the production of cis-urocanic acid in human skin in vivo. J Invest Dermatol. 2005;124(5):1071–4.
17. Ross JA, et al. Ultraviolet irradiated urocanic acid suppresses delayed-type hypersensitivity to herpes simplex in mice. J Invest Dermatol. 1986;87(5):630–3.
18. Norval M. The effect of ultraviolet radiation on human viral infections. Photochem Photobiol. 2006;82(6):1495–504.
19. Jackson S, et al. Role of Bak in UV-induced apoptosis in skin cancer and abrogation by HPV E6 proteins. Genes Dev. 2000;14(23):3065–73.
20. Bedard KM, et al. The E6 oncoproteins from human betapapillomavirus differentially activate telomerase through an E6AP-dependant mechanism and prolong the lifespan of primary keratinocytes. J Virol. 2008;82(8):3894–902.
21. Jensen P, et al. Skin cancer in kidney and heart transplant recipients and different long-term immunosuppressive therapy regimens. J Am Acad Dermatol. 1999;40(2 Pt 1):177–86.
22. Berg D, Otley CC. Skin cancer in organ transplant recipients: epidemiology, pathogenesis, and management. J Am Acad Dermatol. 2002;47:1–17.
23. Finsen NR. Om Bekæmpelse af Lupus vulgaris med en Redegørelse for de i Danmark opnaaede Resultater. Copenhagen: Gyldendalske Boghandels Forlag; 1902.
24. Jones B, Oh C, Corkery E, Hanley R, Egan C. Attitudes and perceptions regarding skin cancer and sun protection behaviour in an Irish population. J Eur Acad Dermatol Venereol. 2007;21:1097–101. doi:10.1111/j.1468-3083.2007.02209.x.
25. Boniol M, et al. Cutaneous melanoma attributable to sunbed use: systematic review and meta-analysis. BMJ. 2012;345:e4757. doi:http://dx.doi.org/10.1136/bmj.e4757. Published 24 July 2012.
26. The Public Health (Sunbeds) Act (12); 2014.
27. Lowe NJ, et al. Low doses of repetitive UVA induce morphologic changes in human skin. J Invest Dermatol. 1995;102(6):739–43.
28. Young AR, et al. The detrimental effects of daily sub-erythemal exposure on human skin in vivo can be prevented by a daily-care broad spectrum sunscreen. J Invest Dermatol. 2007;127:975–8.
29. Green A, et al. Daily sunscreen application and betacarotene supplementation in prevention of basal-cell and squamous-cell carcinomas of the skin: a randomised controlled trial. Lancet. 1999;354(9180):723–9.
30. Thieden E, et al. Ultraviolet exposure patterns of Irish and Danish gardeners during work and leisure. Br J Dermatol. 2005;153:795–801.
31. WHO Global UV project. http://www.who.into/uv/.
32. Gamblicher T, Laperre J, Hoffmann K. The European standard for sun protective clothing: EN13758. J Eur Acad Dermatol Venereol. 2006;20:125–30.
33. Diffey BL. Sun protection with clothing. Br J Dermatol. 2001;144:449–50.
34. Citek K. Anti-reflective coatings reflect ultraviolet radiation. Optometry. 2008;79:143–8.
35. Roberts JE. Ultraviolet radiation as a risk factor for cataract and macular degeneration. Eye Contact Lens. 2011;37(4):246–9.
36. Diffey BL, Cheeseman J. Sun protection with hats. Br J Dermatol. 1992;127(1):10–2.
37. McKinlay AF, Diffey BL. A reference spectrum for ultraviolet induced erythema on human skin. CIE J. 1987;6:17–22.
38. AS/NZS. Australian/New Zealand standard. AS/NZS, 604; 1998.
39. The International Organisation for standardisation. Cosmetics-sun protection test methods-in vivo

determination of the sun protection factor (SPF). ISO 2010; 24444.
40. Diffey BL, Grice J. The influence of sunscreen type on photoprotection. Br J Dermatol. 1997;137:103–5.
41. Nash JF. Human safety and efficacy of ultraviolet filters and sunscreen products. Dermatol Clin. 2006;24:35–51.
42. Azurdia RM, et al. Sunscreen application by photosensitive patients is inadequate for protection. Br J Dermatol. 1999;140:255–8.
43. Faurschou A, Wolf SC. The relation between sun protection factor and the amount of sunscreen applied in vivo. Br J Dermatol. 2007;156:716–9.
44. Rice EG. Dihydroxyacetone naphthoquinone protection against photosensitivity. Dermatalogica. 1976;153:38–43.
45. Faurschou A, Wulf HC. Durability of the sun protection factor provided by dihydroxyacetone. Photodermatol Photoimmunol Photomed. 2004;20(5):239–42.
46. Seite S, Fourtanier AM. The benefit of daily photoprotection. J Am Acad Dermatol. 2008;58(5 Suppl 2):S160–6.
47. Naylor MF, et al. High sun protection factor sunscreens in the suppression of actinic neoplasia. Arch Dermatol. 1995;131:170–5.
48. Lautenschlager S, Wulf HC, Pittelkow MR. Photoprotection. Lancet. 2007;370:528–37.
49. Morales SV, et al. NMSC: an evaluation of risk in terms of UV exposure. Eur J Epidemiol. 1992;8(6):838–44.
50. American Academy of Dermatology. Facts about sunscreens. Schaumburg, Ill: American Academy of Dermatology. http://www.aad.org/media/background/factsheets/fact_sunscreen.htm.
51. Royal D. How to measure UVA protection afforded by sunscreen products. Expert Rev Dermatol. 2008;3(3):307–13.

3 Update on Our Understanding of HPV as a Risk Factor for Cutaneous Squamous Cell Carcinoma in Organ Transplant Recipients

Roel E. Genders, Koen D. Quint, Maurits N.C. de Koning, Elsemieke I. Plasmeijer, Mariet C. Feltkamp, and Jan Nico Bouwes Bavinck

Contents

R.E. Genders, MD • K.D. Quint, MD, PhD
E.I. Plasmeijer, MD, PhD
J.N. Bouwes Bavinck, MD, PhD (✉)
Department of Dermatology, Leiden University Medical Center, Leiden, The Netherlands
e-mail: r.e.genders@lumc.nl; k.d.quint@lumc.nl; e.i.plasmeijer@lumc.nl; J.N.Bouwes_Bavinck@lumc.nl

M.C. Feltkamp, MD, PhD
Department of Medical Microbiology, Leiden University Medical Center, Leiden, The Netherlands
e-mail: m.c.w.feltkamp@lumc.nl

M.N.C. de Koning, PhD
Research and Development, DDL Diagnostic Laboratory, Rijswijk, Zuid Holland, The Netherlands
e-mail: Maurits.dekoning@ddl.nl

3.1 Introduction

3.1.1 Organ Transplant Recipients, Skin Cancer, and Immunosuppressive Therapies

Keratinocyte carcinomas are by far the most common malignancies seen in organ transplant recipients (OTR). The incidence of squamous cell carcinoma (SCC) is 60–250 times increased compared to the immunocompetent population, and for basal cell carcinoma (BCC), this is 10–40 times [1–4].

Lifelong immunosuppressive therapy is the most important risk factor for developing SCC in OTR. Other important risk factors include cumulative sun exposure, smoking, and fair skin type with susceptibility to sunburn, which are risk factors similar to the immunocompetent population [5].

Long-term immunosuppressive therapy predisposes to the development of skin cancer, and

F. Zwald, M.D. Brown (eds.), *Advances in Transplant Dermatology: Clinical and Practical Implications*, DOI 10.1007/978-3-319-12445-2_3, © Springer International Publishing Switzerland 2015

this is related to the type, duration, and intensity of the immunosuppressive therapy. Azathioprine increases the photosensitivity of human skin to UVA radiation, and when exposed to UVA radiation, the active metabolite, methyl-thioinosine monophosphate (MeTIMP), which is incorporated into cellular DNA, generates reactive mutagenic oxygen species [6, 7]. The carcinogenic effect of calcineurin inhibitors (cyclosporine and tacrolimus) is linked to aberrant production of cytokines that promote tumor growth, metastasis, and angiogenesis [8].

Immunosuppressive therapy with mammalian target of rapamycin (mTOR) inhibitors is possibly associated with a reduced risk of cutaneous SCC by antitumor and antiangiogenic properties, but seems only effective when the number of SCC is still low and during the first year after conversion to mTOR inhibitor [9–11].

3.1.2 Human Papillomavirus Infection

Human papillomaviruses (HPV) cause several distinct benign and (pre-)malignant diseases. HPV can be divided into alpha, beta, gamma, mu, and nu genera. Well-known associations with benign lesions are with common skin warts (verruca vulgaris) and genital warts (condyloma accuminata). The most prevalent HPV types associated with common warts are the Alpha-PV types 2, 27, and 57 and the Gamma-PV type 4 [12–14]. The majority of genital warts are caused by the mucosal Alpha-PV types 6 and 11, but other mucosal HPV types of the alpha genera are also detected in genital warts.

The range of infections, precancers, and malignancies associated with HPV continues to grow. The International Agency for Research on Cancer (IARC) has classified mucosal types 16, 18, 31, 33, 35, 39, 45, 51, 52, 56, 58, and 59 as carcinogenic types (Class 1), mainly causing cervical cancer; type 68 as probably carcinogenic (Class 2A); and types 26, 30, 34, 53, 66, 67, 69, 70, 73, 82, 85, and 97 as possibly carcinogenic (Class 2B). HPV6 and HPV11 were not classifiable as to its carcinogenicity to humans, and the remaining mucosal HPV types were not taken into consideration by IARC (Class 3) [15].

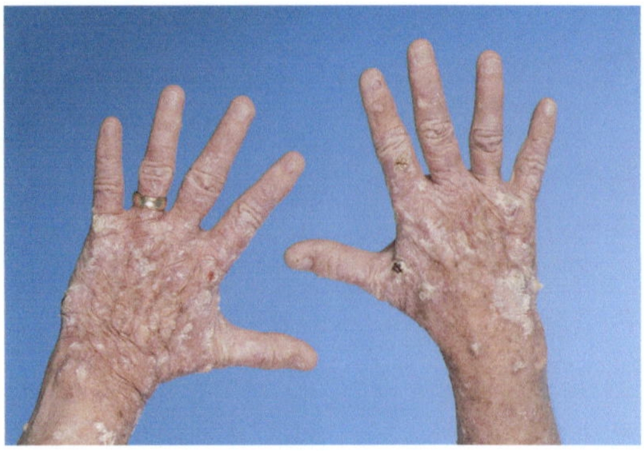

Fig. 3.1 Multiple wartlike lesions on dorsum of the hands

The first time that HPV infection was linked with skin cancer was in patients with epidermodysplasia verruciformis (EV). EV is a rare autosomal recessive disease, initially described by Lewandowsky and Lutz in 1922, that has been proposed as a model for Beta-PV-mediated skin carcinogenesis [16]. EV patients have an increased susceptibility to widespread Beta-PV infections of the skin and develop pityriasis versicolor-like lesions and flat warts [17, 18]. Skin cancers develop in one-third of the patients, mainly on sun-exposed sites in young to middle-aged adult patients [19].

In the years after transplantation, OTR develop numerous warts and wartlike lesions followed by the development of SCC (Figs. 3.1 and 3.2), which resembles the clinical picture of EV patients. The association between wartlike lesions and SCC in OTR is an argument that HPV infection may play a role in SCC carcinogenesis [20, 21]. This chapter will further focus on Beta-PV infection as a possible risk factor for cutaneous SCC carcinogenesis in OTR. In the following paragraphs laboratory and epidemiological evidence linking HPV infection with the development of SCC will be discussed. The HPV genome and taxonomy, replication and influence on cell cycle, and Beta-PV detection methods will be covered as well.

3.2 Human Papillomaviruses

3.2.1 HPV Genome and Taxonomy

Papillomaviruses (PV) are nonenveloped circular double-stranded DNA viruses belonging to the family *papillomaviridae*. The genome is approximately 8 kb and slightly varies in size between types. More than 150 types have been identified today, and the number is still increasing (Fig. 3.3). The genome is subdivided in an early (E) coding region, a late (L) coding region, and a long control region (LCR). The early region generally encodes for six nonstructural viral regulatory proteins (E1, E2, E4, E5, E6, and E7 in most PV types and an additional E8 in some PV types) involved in several functions including transformation, transcription, and viral adaptation to different cellular milieus [23]. The late region encodes for two structural proteins, namely, L1 and L2 [24]. Whereas all PV appear to have an E1, E2, L1, and L2 open reading frame (ORF), the other ORFs are not consistently present in every PV [13]. Beta-PV have E1, E2, E4, E6, E7, L1, and L2 ORFs, but lack E5.

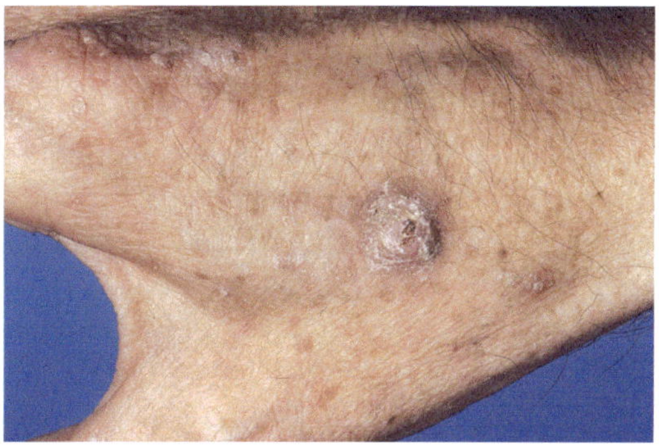

Fig. 3.2 Squamous cell carcinoma on dorsum of the hand

The L1 ORF encoding for the major capsid protein L1 is relatively well conserved between HPV types. The L1 protein is the basis for currently registered prophylactic vaccines against

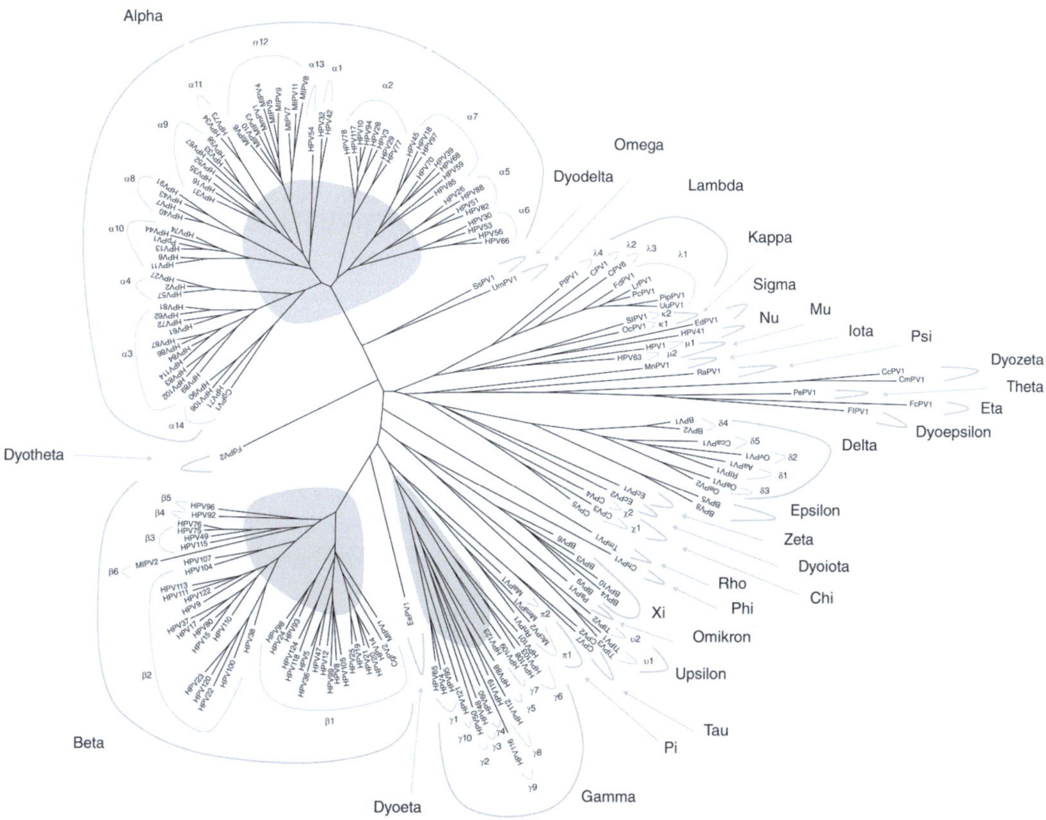

Fig. 3.3 Phylogenetic tree (Modified from Bernard et al. [22])

Table 3.1 HPV types sorted by genus

Genus	HPV type
Alpha	2, 3, 6, 7, 10, 11, 13, 16,18, 26, 27, 28, 29, 30, 31, 32, 33, 34, 35, 39, 40, 42, 43, 44, 45, 51, 52, 53, 54, 55, 56, 57, 58, 59, 61, 62, 66, 67, 68, 69, 70, 71, 72, 73, 74, 77, 78, 81, 82, 83, 84, 85, 86, 87, 89, 90, 91, 94, 97, 102, 106, 114, 117, 125, 160
Beta	5, 8, 9, 12, 14, 15, 17, 19, 20, 21, 22, 23, 24, 25, 36, 37, 38, 47, 49, 75, 76, 80, 92, 93, 96, 98, 99, 100, 104, 105, 107, 110, 111, 113, 115, 118, 120, 122, 124, 143, 145, 150, 151, 159
Gamma	4, 48, 50, 60, 65, 88, 95, 101, 103, 108, 109, 112, 116, 119, 121, 123, 126, 127, 128, 129, 130, 131, 132, 133, 134, 135, 136, 137, 138, 139, 140, 141, 142, 144, 146, 147, 148, 149, 153, 154, 155, 156, 161, 162, 163, 164, 165, 166, 169, 170
Mu	1, 63
Nu	41

Source: http://pave.niaid.nih.gov/#home

HPV types 6, 11, 16, and 18 infections that cause genital warts and cervical cancer. The current papillomavirus classification system is based on DNA sequence homology of the L1 ORF and comprises a division in genus, species, type, subtype, and variants. The phylogenetic tree is shown in Fig. 3.3 [22].

As stated before, HPV can be divided into alpha, beta, gamma, mu, and nu genera. Species of the same genera share at least 60 % homology of the L1 ORF. A new type is defined as one in which the complete nucleotide sequence ORF of the L1 gene differs by more than 10 % from the most closely related known PV type. Table 3.1 shows all the HPV types according to the genus, based on the Papillomavirus Episteme database (http://pave.niaid.nih.gov/#home). The beta, gamma, mu, and nu genera are cutaneous types. The alpha genus contains all the mucosal types but also some cutaneous types (HPV2, 3, 10, 27, 28, 29, 57, 77, 94) and mucocutaneous types (HPV7, 40, 43, 91) [22].

3.2.2 HPV Life Cycle

HPV infection occurs when the virus enters the basal layer of the epithelium, supposedly achieved by small abrasions of the epithelium. However, the body-wide distribution of especially Beta-PV infections suggests a direct route of infection, bypassing the requirement of epithelial injury or abrasion [25–29]. Life cycle studies have been mainly performed for the HPV types causing cervical cancer, but the life cycle of several HPV types with a cutaneous tropism appears to be similar [30].

E6 and E7 are mainly expressed in the (supra) basal layer and the granular layer of the epithelium and are associated with PV genome maintenance and cellular proliferation. E1 and E2 are involved in viral DNA replication and the regulation of E6 and E7 transcription. E4 of some cutaneous HPV types appears to be expressed throughout the epithelium except in the basal cell layer [31] and presumably promotes viral DNA replication [32]. There is some variability in viral life cycle between PV types. However, the order of expression of viral genes throughout the differentiating epithelia is similar, although the localization of E4 and L1 expression is variable and starts either in the lower part of the epithelium (HPV1 and 2) or in the upper part (HPV63 and 65) [33].

3.2.3 Beta-PV Detection Methods

There are different methods for Beta-PV detection, based on measurement of viral protein, viral DNA, or serum antibody responses. Tissue specimens can be collected via several sampling methods like skin swabs, plucked hairs, biopsies, and blood [34]. Several PCR-based methods targeting the HPV L1, E1, or E7 ORF have been developed to detect Beta-PV types in skin biopsies, plucked hairs, and skin swabs [25, 26, 35–45].

These PCR methods can be divided into (I) type-specific PCRs, using HPV type-specific primers for the detection of a single HPV type; (II) multiplex type-specific PCR methods, in which multiple type-specific primer sets are combined in a single PCR reaction; (III) broad-spectrum PCR methods using consensus primers, which permit simultaneous amplification of multiple types; and (IV) quantitative PCR methods that allow viral DNA quantification.

Multiplex type-specific PCR and broad-spectrum PCR–based methods amplify multiple HPV types in a single reaction. Subsequent genotyping in the case of amplification systems that target multiple HPV types is generally performed by sequence analysis, either directly or preceded by cloning of the amplimer. Sequencing, however, does not easily permit the identification of HPV types present in frequently occurring multiple infections [39, 46]. Therefore, the more recently developed PCRs are followed by reverse hybridization technologies or APEX for the simultaneous identification of multiple HPV types [39, 41, 45, 47].

With viruslike particle (VLP) enzyme-linked immunoassay (ELISA) or multiplex technology (Luminex), antibodies against Beta-PV viral proteins can be detected, to determine a person's Beta-PV serological status. Serologic responses are usually measured against the major capsid protein L1 and the nonstructural protein E6 using HPV viruslike particle (VLP) or GST-HPV fusion proteins in ELISA [48, 49] or with multiplex serology using GST-L1 fusion proteins, respectively [50]. The latter method (Luminex) is based on fluorescent bead technology that allows simultaneous detection of antibodies against up to 100 different in situ affinity-purified recombinant HPV proteins [51]. However, not all HPV infections induce an antibody response to HPV, and cross-reactive antibodies between different HPV types may be produced [52]. Nevertheless, serologic antibody responses provide a useful epidemiologic tool to explore HPV infections in certain populations.

Detection of papillomavirus proteins and DNA in paraffin-embedded tissue sections is possible by combining in situ hybridization and fluorescence detection methods (FISH = Fluorescent DNA in situ hybridization) [53]. Also laser capture microdissection can be used to specifically test a particular part of a histological specimen for HPV presence and viral load [54].

3.2.4 Beta-PV Replication, Cell Transformation, and Carcinogenesis

After infection, Beta-PV will start to replicate in the epidermal keratinocytes. As for mucosal HPV, keratinocyte differentiation is probably also crucial for Beta-PV to fulfill their life cycle [55, 56]. It is expected that in the basal epidermal layers a low level of replication of Beta-PV DNA is maintained to ensure viral episome distribution among daughter cells, and especially the early (E) genes will be expressed [57].

Transformation of human cells has been studied in great detail for the HPV types causing cervical cancer (e.g., HPV16 and HPV18). In general, transformation requires long-term and deregulated expression of viral oncogenes E6 and E7. This process is facilitated by integration of the viral episome into the cellular DNA, disturbing the E2 ORF, thereby causing a lack of control of E6 and E7 expression [32]. In general, Beta-PV are found episomal, also in actinic keratoses and SCC, although (integrated) HPV has been occasionally isolated from an SCC metastatic lesion in an OTR [43, 58].

Since papillomaviruses depend on (unscheduled) host cell DNA replication in order to produce progeny, the virus tends to keep its host cell in a replicative state (S-phase) as long as possible. This is particularly relevant as terminal keratinocyte differentiation is a dead-end road resembling programmed cell death (apoptosis) [59, 60]. For high-risk mucosal HPV types, it is known that the E7 early gene product drives cells into S phase by binding and degrading the tumor suppressor protein pRb [61]. For HPV38, a Beta-PV type that has been associated with SCC in some studies, this has been shown as well, but it does not seem to be a mechanism exploited by all Beta-PV types. For the high-risk mucosal HPVs, such as HPV16 and HPV18, this mechanism acts through ubiquitination and subsequent degradation of the tumor suppressors p53 and pRb. Presumably, persistent infections are needed to accumulate sufficient mutations in the host cellular genome to generate a malignant cell. The proliferative phenotype of these malignant cells remains dependent on E6/E7 expression [62].

HPV38 E7 was shown to bind and degrade the tumor suppressor pRb similar as HPV16 E7 [63, 64]. Furthermore, HPV38 E6 and E7 are sufficient to deregulate the cell cycle and senescence programs in primary human keratinocytes, thereby increasing the lifespan of human skin keratinocytes [63, 65, 66]. HPV38 E6, possibly in combination with E7, induces telomerase activity, which plays a key role in transformation of human keratinocytes [67].

Another mechanism behind the lack of cell cycle arrest in Beta-PV expressing cells might be the upregulation of delta-Np73 as a result of p53 accumulation [68, 69]. This upregulation prevents p53 to induce the transcription of genes involved in apoptosis and growth suppression, altering the regulation of cell cycle checkpoints that are normally activated by UV radiation [69].

Several studies investigating the effect of Beta-PV E6 and E7 in organotypic (raft) cultures showed that Beta-PV could delay cell differentiation and disturb keratinocyte outgrowth [66, 70–72].

As the vast majority of SCC occurs on sun-exposed sites, it is generally believed that Beta-PV, if involved in skin cancer development, somehow cooperates with UV radiation in transforming cutaneous epithelial keratinocytes. Beta-PV could confer its possible carcinogenic effect via inhibition of DNA repair and apoptosis in UV-damaged cells which is illustrated in Fig. 3.4 [73].

HPV5 E6 appeared to exert this effect via the degradation of Bak, a protein involved in induction of apoptosis [74–76]. The E6 of HPV8, 20, 22, 38, 76, 92, and 96 can protect UV-treated keratinocytes from apoptosis [77, 78]. The oncoproteins E6 and E7 from Beta-PV38 significantly contribute to SCC development in the skin rendering keratinocytes more susceptible to UV-induced carcinogenesis in mice [79, 80]. Interference with UV-induced DNA repair and apoptosis by Beta-PV might occur, and epidemiological studies seem suggestive of a joint effect of UV radiation and Beta-PV infection as well [50, 73, 81].

Still other studies have shown that the E6 proteins of HPV5 and HPV8 inhibit the transforming growth factor beta (TGF-beta) signaling pathway by the degradation of the SMAD3 transcription factor [82]. TGF-beta-triggered pathways lead to the synthesis of inhibitors (p16, p17, p21, and p27) of the cyclin-dependent kinases that play a crucial role in the cell cycle. It can be postulated that specific degradation of SMAD3 could negatively regulate inhibitors of the cell cycle and favor cell transition from the G1 to the S phase, allowing viral DNA vegetative replication and, as a side effect, cell transformation.

Additionally, there is evidence that the association of HPV5 and HPV8 E6 proteins with MAML1 inhibits Notch signaling and that Notch signaling plays a role in both virus–host perturbations and tumor genesis [83].

In HPV-positive skin cancers, not all tumor cells contain HPV DNA, and the viral load is higher in actinic keratoses [84]. If Beta-PV are involved in the development of skin cancer, they probably play a role in tumor initiation and progression, not in maintenance of the malignant phenotype, through a "hit-and-run" mechanism of viral carcinogenesis [79].

3.3 Epidemiology of HPV Infection and Skin Cancer

3.3.1 HPV Carriage in Humans

HPV DNA can frequently be detected in skin swabs and plucked hairs in newborns, children, and adults [29, 34, 50, 85–89]. Family members may share some of the same HPV types [29, 90]. The prevalence of HPV DNA ranges between 42 and 87 %, and 84 and 91 %, respectively, using skin swab and plucked hair sampling, and varies also between geographical regions and ethnicities [25, 29, 46, 90–95].

Viral DNA is persistent in/on the skin [86, 89, 95]. Increasing age, sun exposure, sunburn, skin type, and a medical history of skin cancer are factors which are associated with an increased prevalence of HPV DNA [4, 25, 91, 96, 97]. Duration of immunosuppression and immunosuppression itself in OTR is also associated with an increased prevalence of HPV DNA

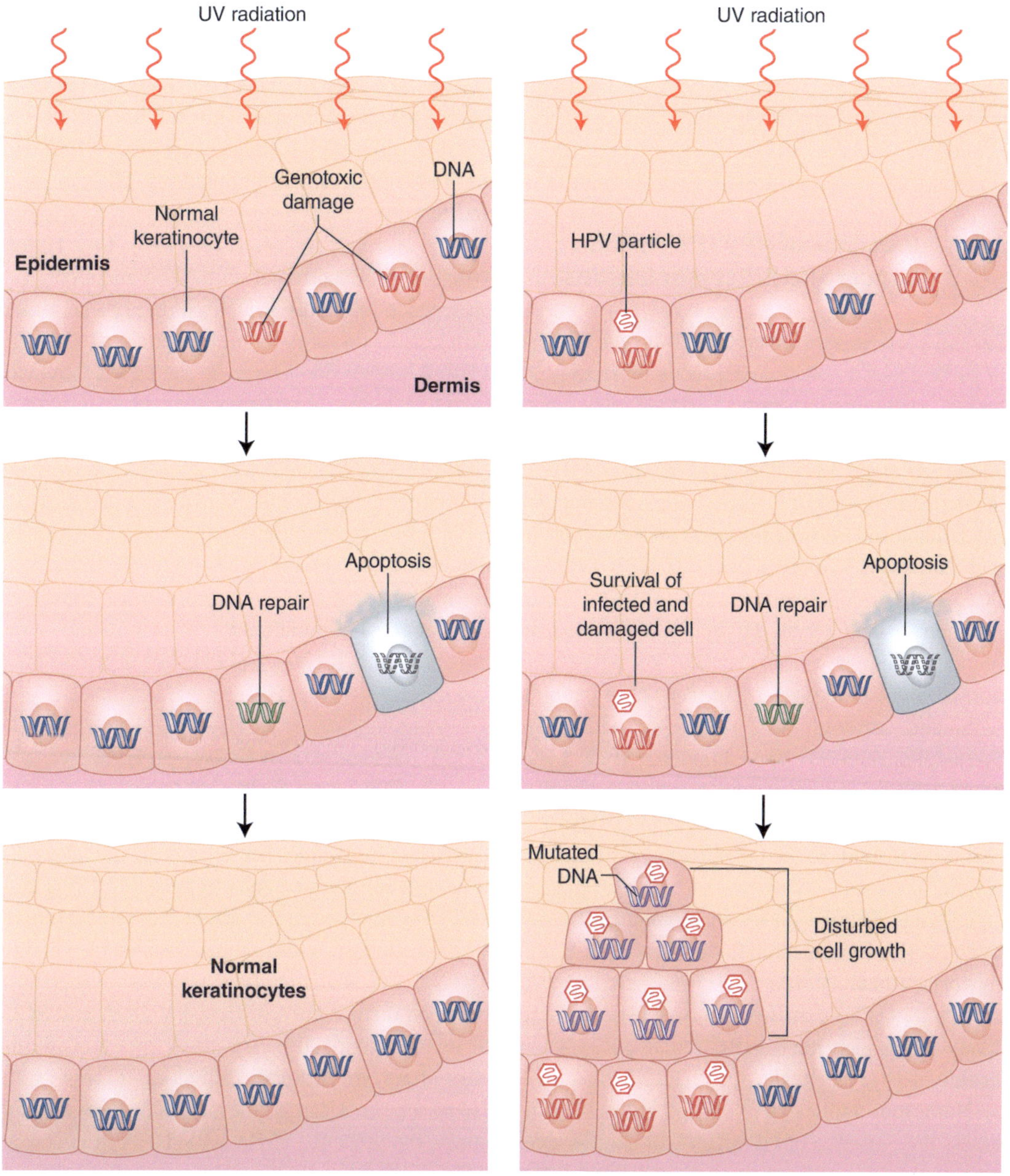

Fig. 3.4 Ultraviolet radiation causes genotoxic damage in the keratinocytes in the basal layer of the epidermis. Panels on the *left* illustrate DNA repair in the cells or dying due to apoptosis. The panels on the *right* show the situation when a keratinocyte is infected with HPV. The infected keratinocyte has low ability for DNA repair and is less sensitive to apoptosis. The DNA mutated cell can proliferate and multiply and lead to dysplastic keratinocytes. Currently it is believed that not every mutated cell carries a virus episome (Permission for reprint accepted by *NEJM* (rights JNBB))

in plucked hair samples compared with the immunocompetent population [46].

Seropositivity for one or more HPV types is approximately 60 % in the general population (most frequently for HPV 8 followed by HPV 15, 17, 38, and 49), but can be higher in certain subpopulations [97–99]. Serological responses to HPV are also more common in OTR and vary between 80 and 90 % to at least one HPV type. Between 45 and 56 % of these positive seroresponses are against Beta-PV types. Most commonly detected Beta-PV types are HPV 8, 15, 17, 38, and 49 [25, 100, 101].

3.3.2 Presence of HPV DNA in Skin Cancer and Precursor Lesions

Several studies have investigated the prevalence of HPV DNA in SCC and precursor lesions in both immunocompetent individuals and OTR. HPV carriage was nicely summarized by Aldabagh et al. [34]. The percentages of HPV DNA positivity vary between immunocompetent individuals and OTR and depend on the detection methods used. The prevalences of HPV DNA in SCC in the immunocompetent population range between 26 and 69 %. HPV DNA can also be found in benign lesions, actinic keratosis, and normal and sun-exposed skin from both patients with and without SCC [84, 94, 102–105]. Frequently, Beta-PV types, including HPV 5 and 8, are detected in higher rates in actinic keratoses compared to SCC [106]. Viral load of HPV infection was found to be significantly higher in actinic keratoses compared to SCC [84]. In a small study Beta-PV DNA was found to be more often present in perilesional skin than in SCC and mirror site healthy skin [107], but there are also studies reporting that Beta-PV species 2 is more likely to be identified in SCC than in adjacent healthy skin [102, 103].

Numerous studies were carried out in OTR to assess the presence of HPV DNA in keratinocyte carcinomas. De Villiers et al. found HPV DNA positivity in 91 % of SCC and in situ SCC in 25 OTR, the most prevalent types being among the Beta-PV types [38]. Berkhout et al. found similar frequencies and distribution of Beta-PV types in hyperkeratotic papillomas, actinic keratosis, and SCC, but lower in BCC, benign lesions, and normal skin [108].

Some studies have compared the prevalence of HPV DNA in SCC and precursor lesions of immunocompetent individuals with OTR. In a German study, HPV DNA was detected more frequently in SCC of OTR (75 %) than in immunocompetent patients (47 %) [109]. Similar HPV prevalences were found in cutaneous warts (91 % vs. 94 %), premalignant skin tumors (38 % vs. 36 %), and normal skin specimens (17 % vs. 16 %) for both patient populations. HPV types 5 and 8 were found more frequently in SCCs and only in the SCC of the OTR [109]. In a Dutch group of OTR with and without skin cancer, the prevalence of Beta-PV DNA in benign keratotic skin lesions was equally high, around 50 % [108–110]. A higher prevalence of Beta-PV DNA was found in lesions from sun-exposed sites with a history of skin cancer [110]. In a Scottish study no difference was detected between lesions from immunocompetent individuals and OTR with HPV 15, 24, and 38 as the most frequently detected types. In this study multiple infections were more common in tumors from immunocompetent individuals (70 %) compared with those from OTR (26 %) [111].

3.3.3 Association Between HPV DNA and Skin Cancer

Case–control studies investigating the association between the presence of Beta-PV DNA and SCC are summarized in Table 3.2. Most studies were performed with immunocompetent patients and show a statistically significant association between the presence of Beta-PV DNA and SCC or its precursor actinic keratoses, or a nonsignificant trend in the same direction (Table 3.2). However, in a large international case–control study, the presence of Beta-PV DNA in eyebrow hairs was only significantly associated with an increased risk of SCC in the Netherlands, but not in Italy and Australia [87]. Overall the Beta-PV DNA positivity was more than 90 % for all participants [87]. So far, only one large study was performed with European OTR showing a 2.4 times increased risk of SCC in OTR with Beta-PV DNA in eyebrow hairs [116].

High viral load of Beta-PV DNA in eyebrow hairs was reported to be associated with increased risk of cutaneous SCC in immunocompetent Australian patients and in OTR, with total load

Table 3.2 Epidemiological studies summarizing the association between Beta-PV DNA and SCC development

Author (Ref.)	Study type	Population/ country	Infection marker	Method	HPV types	Cases	Controls	Adjusted odds ratio (95 % CI)	Comments
Boxman et al. [36]	Nested case–control	IC/Australia	DNA in eyebrow hairs	Nested PCR	Beta	64 KC* 51 BCC 25 SCC	64 51 25	0.8 (0.3–1.8) 0.6 (0.2–1.5) 2.0 (0.5–8.0)	*BCC/SCC/intraepithelial carcinoma/KC undefined
Boxman et al. [112]	Cross sectional	IC/Australia	DNA in eyebrow hairs	Nested PCR	Beta	276 AK	231	3.4 (1.8–6.5) (M) 1.0 (0.6–1.8) (F)	Significant association between Beta-PV and AK only in men
Struijk et al. [113]	Case–control	IC/the Netherlands	DNA in eyebrow hairs	Type-specific PCR	2, 5, 8, 15, 16, 20, 24, 38	155 SCC	371	1.7 (1.1–2.7)	Association between Beta-PV and SCC with increasing age and male sex
Harwood et al. [114]	Case–control	IC/UK	DNA in normal skin biopsies	Degenerate/nested PCR	Beta	10 KC*	29	6.4 (1.8–22.9)	*BCC/SCC
Struijk et al. [49]	Case–control	IC/Australia	DNA in eyebrow hairs	Type-specific PCR	5, 8, 15, 20, 24, 38	126 AK 64 SCC	57	1.6 (0.8–3.0) 0.9 (0.4–2.0)	
McBride et al. [115]	Prospective	IC/Australia	DNA in eyebrow hairs	Nested PCR	Beta	71 (1–10) AK 41 > 10 AK	179	1.8 (0.7–4.4)	Association with having more than 10 AK. Significant associations with age over 60 years, fair skin color, high sun exposure
Bouwes Bavinck et al. [87]	Case–control	IC/Australia (AU), Italy (I), the Netherlands (NL)	DNA in eyebrow hairs	PCR–reverse hybridization assay	Beta	689 SCC	845	2.8 (1.3–5.8) NL 1.7 (0.79–3.6) I 0.91 (0.53–1.6) AU	
Proby et al. [116]	Case–control	IS/France, Italy, the Netherlands, UK	DNA in eyebrow hairs	PCR–reverse hybridization assay	Beta	210 SCC	394	2.4 (1–5.4)	For HPV5, 9, 24, and 36

IC immunocompetent, *IS* immunosuppressed/transplant patients, *KC* keratinocyte cancer, *AK* actinic keratosis, *BCC* basal cell carcinoma, *SCC* squamous cell carcinoma seemingly more important than the load of any specific type [117].

Exposure to individual cutaneous HPV types and the risk of SCC was recently summarized [118]. Many Beta-PV types are associated with an increased risk of SCC, but no specific type stands out. HPV 9, 24, 36, 76, and 92 showed the strongest association with SCC [118].

With respect to the presence of Beta-PV DNA in (pre-)malignant and benign skin tumors, no correlation was found with serum antibodies to the same HPV type measured. However, seropositivity to any HPV type was significantly more common among patients positive for HPV DNA of any HPV type, and seroprevalences were higher for SCC patients compared to BCC patients [85].

3.3.4 Association Between HPV Serology and Skin Cancer

Most studies investigating the association between serologic antibody responses to HPV and SCC were also carried out in the immunocompetent population and show a statistically significant association between the presence of Beta-PV antibodies and SCC, or a nonsignificant trend in the same direction (Tables 3.2 and 3.3). The odds ratios are increasing when there are more positive serological responses against increasing numbers of Beta-PV types [48, 50, 121, 124, 125]. The association with SCC is exclusively found for Beta-PV types, particularly HPV 5, 8, 9, 15, 17, 20, 24, 36, 38, 49, 75, 76, and 92, but not for Alpha-, Gamma-, Mu-, or Nu-PV types [118].

In an international case–control study, a positive antibody response against 4 or more Beta-PV types was associated with a doubled risk for SCC in Australia and the Netherlands [87]. A population-based cohort study in Australia, however, revealed no associations between the presence of any Beta-PV antibodies and the occurrence of SCC. However, among people who were less than 50 years old in 1992, the presence of Beta-PV antibodies was associated with a twofold increased risk of SCC [126]. In the United Kingdom in a prospective pilot study among 39 SCC cases and 80 controls, also no statistically significant differences were found in the seroprevalence of antibodies against any of 38 HPV types [128]. HPV seropositivity was strongly associated with the risk of developing a second SCC after 5 years for both Beta-PV and Gamma-PV types [127].

3.3.5 Viral Transcriptional Activity and Skin Cancer

Viral transcriptional activity was investigated in SCC from both immunocompetent individuals and OTR. Only a portion of SCC was positive for cutaneous HPV using in situ hybridization [129], but similarly low transcriptional activity in warts in OTR was observed [129]. The biological activity of HPV types found in tumor tissues was assessed by examining HPV E6/E7 RNA expression for cutaneous HPV types. HPV DNA was detected in 25 of 31 tissue samples. E6/E7 transcripts of HPV 8, 9, and 15 were found in low copy numbers in one SCC and three AKs, but not in normal skin or verrucae vulgaris [130].

Transcriptome sequencing, performed on 31 SCCs, failed to identify HPV expression in any of the skin tumors [131].

3.3.6 Human Papillomavirus and Basal Cell Carcinoma

A recent systematic review showed no association between Beta-PV DNA or Beta-PV serological responses and BCC [118]. In a subgroup of patients with Beta-PV DNA-positive BCC, however, an association between a serological response against Beta-PV and BCC could be observed [132]. Some Beta-PV types could upregulate the p16^{INK4a} and Akt/P13K pathway and might play a role in the carcinogenesis of BCC [133]. The evidence that HPV is involved in BCC carcinogenesis is clearly much weaker than the possible involvement of HPV in cutaneous SCC carcinogenesis.

Table 3.3 Epidemiological studies summarizing the association between Beta-PV seroprevalence and SCC development

Author (Ref.)	Study type	Population/ country	Infection marker	Method	HPV types	Cases	Controls	Adjusted odds ratio (95 % CI)	Comments
Steger et al. [119]	Case–control	IC/Germany	L1 serology	Western blot	8	11	445	10.7 (2.5–63.2)	
Stark et al. [120]	Case–control	IC/Germany	L1 serology	ELISA	8	14 SCC	210	30.3 (7.4–142.5)	
Bouwes Bavinck et al. [121]	Case–control	IC/the Netherlands	L1 serology	ELISA	8	13 SCC	82	3.1 (0.7–13.3)	
Feltkamp et al. [48]	Case–control/ Netherlands	IC/the Netherlands	L1 serology	ELISA	5, 8, 15, 20, 24, 38	540 SCC	333	1.4 (0.8–2.5)	
Masini et al. [122]	Case–control	IC/Italy	L1 serology	ELISA	8, 15, 23, 36	46 SCC	84	3.2 (1.3–7.9) (HPV8) 0.4 (0.2–0.9) (HPV15) 1.0 (0.3–3.3) (HPV23) 2.8 (0.8–10.0) (HPV36)	
Karagas et al. [50]	Case–control	IC/USA	L1 serology	Multiplex	Beta	252 SCC	461	1.5 (1.1–2.1)	
Struijk et al. [49]	Case–control	IC/Australia	L1/E6 serology	ELISA	5, 8, 15, 16, 20, 24, 38	126 AK 64 SCC	57	2.3 (0.9–4.9)(L1) 0.6 (0.3–1.3) (E6) 3.9 (1.4–10.7) (L1) 0.5 (0.2–1.1) (E6)	Associations between Beta-PV L1 and E6 serology and AK/SCC
Casabonne et al. [123]	Nested case–control	IC/UK	L1 serology	Multiplex	Beta	39 SCC	80	0.5 (0.1–1.7)* 1.0 (0.4–2.5) **	Association between 1* or 2+** Beta-PV type(s) and SCC
Karagas et al. [124]	Case–control	IC/USA	L1 serology	Multiplex	Beta	663 SCC	805	1.0 (0.7–1.3)* 1.4 (1.0–2.0)** 1.5 (1.0–2.2)*** 1.7 (1.1–2.6)****	Association between 1* or 2–3**, 4–8***, or >8**** Beta-PV type(s) and SCC
Proby et al. [116]	Case–control	IS/France, Italy, the Netherlands, UK	L1 serology	Multiplex	Beta	210 SCC	394	1.6 (1.1–2.5)	Association for concordant detection of both antibodies and DNA for at least one Beta-PV type

(continued)

Table 3.3 (continued)

Author (Ref.)	Study type	Population/ country	Infection marker	Method	HPV types	Cases	Controls	Adjusted odds ratio (95 % CI)	Comments
Waterboer et al. [125]	Case–control	IC/Italy	L1 serology	Multiplex	Beta/Gamma	43 SCC	77	2.8 (1.1–7.1)* 2.6 (1.0–6.5)** 3.0 (1.2–7.9)*** 3.4 (1.2–9.5)****	*HPV15 **HPV17 ***HPV38 ****HPV50
Bouwes Bavinck et al. [87]	Case–control	IC/Australia (AU), Italy (I), the Netherlands (NL)	L1 serology	Multiplex	Beta	689 SCC	845	>=4 types positive 2.0 (1.2–3.4)* 2.2 (1.4–3.3)** 1.6 (0.94–2.7)***	*NL **AU ***I fair skinned
Plasmeijer et al. [126]	Prospective	IC/Australia	L1 serology	Multiplex	Beta	150 SCC	1,161	1.0 (0.7–1.4)* 2.1 (1.0–4.6)**	*HR for being positive for at least 1 Beta-PV type **HR in subset of people <50y
Paradisi et al. [127]	Case–control	IC/Italy	L1 serology	Multiplex	Beta/Gamma	16 SCC	48	4.25 (1.22–15.58)* 8.08 (1.05–62.42)** 3.01 (1.01–8.97)*** 3.46 (1.08–11.5)****	*HR HPV24 **HR HPV15 ***HR HPV95 ****HR HPV60

IC immunocompetent, *IS* immunosuppressed/transplant patients, *KC* keratinocyte cancer, *AK* actinic keratosis, *BCC* basal cell carcinoma, *SCC* squamous cell carcinoma

Conclusions

The role of Beta-PV in cutaneous SCC carcinogenesis is still enigmatic and clearly different from the role of mucosal Alpha-PV types in cervical cancer. Despite experimental evidence and a plausible hypothesis of a biological mechanism supporting a carcinogenic role of Beta-PV in SCC carcinogenesis, the epidemiological studies are still difficult to interpret. The viral load and the plurality of Beta-PV types are an important obstacle to identify the responsible HPV types in epidemiological studies. Several case–control studies observed an association between Beta-PV antibodies in the serum and/or Beta-PV DNA in plucked eyebrow hairs and development of cutaneous SCC, but so far no specific high-risk Beta-PV types could be identified. Possibly much larger studies will be needed to identify the responsible HPV types in between the massive number of bystander HPV types. It is also not clear what the implications are in daily practice for Beta-PV infections in OTR.

Since Beta-PV is not integrated in the human cellular DNA and is not necessary for the maintenance of the malignant phenotype of cutaneous SCC, the carcinogenic effect, if present, is subtle and probably exerted early in carcinogenesis. This fits with observations that premalignant lesions such as actinic keratoses often contain a higher load of Beta-PV compared to SCC. By impairing DNA repair and UV-induced apoptosis, these persistent skin viruses may, after a long period, lead to cellular instability and sequentially cause field changes, actinic keratoses, and finally cutaneous SCC. Whether different Beta-PV types have different effects on cellular mechanisms and a combination of these HPV types may further increase the risk of cutaneous SCC is unknown. Further research is clearly needed to unravel the secrets of Beta-PV in SCC carcinogenesis.

References

1. Euvrard S, Kanitakis J, Claudy A. Skin cancers after organ transplantation. N Engl J Med. 2003;348(17):1681–91.
2. Hartevelt MM, Bavinck JN, Kootte AM, Vermeer BJ, Vandenbroucke JP. Incidence of skin cancer after renal transplantation in The Netherlands. Transplantation. 1990;49(3):506–9.
3. Moloney FJ, Comber H, O'Lorcain P, O'Kelly P, Conlon PJ, Murphy GM. A population-based study of skin cancer incidence and prevalence in renal transplant recipients. Br J Dermatol. 2006;154(3):498–504.
4. Tessari G, Naldi L, Boschiero L, Nacchia F, Fior F, Forni A, et al. Incidence and clinical predictors of a subsequent nonmelanoma skin cancer in solid organ transplant recipients with a first nonmelanoma skin cancer: a multicenter cohort study. Arch Dermatol. 2010;146(3):294–9.
5. Terhorst D, Drecoll U, Stockfleth E, Ulrich C. Organ transplant recipients and skin cancer: assessment of risk factors with focus on sun exposure. Br J Dermatol. 2009;161 Suppl 3:85–9.
6. O'Donovan P, Perrett CM, Zhang X, Montaner B, Xu YZ, Harwood CA, et al. Azathioprine and UVA light generate mutagenic oxidative DNA damage. Science. 2005;309(5742):1871–4.
7. Perrett CM, Walker SL, O'Donovan P, Warwick J, Harwood CA, Karran P, et al. Azathioprine treatment photosensitizes human skin to ultraviolet A radiation. Br J Dermatol. 2008;159(1):198–204.
8. Guba M, Graeb C, Jauch KW, Geissler EK. Pro- and anti-cancer effects of immunosuppressive agents used in organ transplantation. Transplantation. 2004;77(12):1777–82.
9. Euvrard S, Morelon E, Rostaing L, Goffin E, Brocard A, Tromme I, et al. Sirolimus and secondary skin-cancer prevention in kidney transplantation. N Engl J Med. 2012;367(4):329–39.
10. Hoogendijk-van den Akker JM, Harden PN, Hoitsma AJ, Proby CM, Wolterbeek R, Bouwes Bavinck JN, et al. Two-year randomized controlled prospective trial converting treatment of stable renal transplant recipients with cutaneous invasive squamous cell carcinomas to sirolimus. J Clin Oncol. 2013;31(10):1317–23.
11. Kauffman HM, Cherikh WS, Cheng Y, Hanto DW, Kahan BD. Maintenance immunosuppression with target-of-rapamycin inhibitors is associated with a reduced incidence of de novo malignancies. Transplantation. 2005;80(7):883–9.
12. Bruggink SC, de Koning MN, Gussekloo J, Egberts PF, Ter SJ, Feltkamp MC, et al. Cutaneous wart-associated HPV types: prevalence and relation with patient characteristics. J Clin Virol. 2012;55(3):250–5.
13. de Villiers EM, Fauquet C, Broker TR, Bernard HU, zur Hausen H. Classification of papillomaviruses. Virology. 2004;324(1):17–27.
14. Jablonska S, Orth G, Obalek S, Croissant O. Cutaneous warts. Clinical, histologic, and virologic correlations. Clin Dermatol. 1985;3(4):71–82.
15. Bouvard V, Baan R, Straif K, Grosse Y, Secretan B, El GF, et al. A review of human carcinogens–Part B: biological agents. Lancet Oncol. 2009;10(4):321–2.
16. Jablonska S, Dabrowski J, Jakubowicz K. Epidermodysplasia verruciformis as a model in

studies on the role of papovaviruses in oncogenesis. Cancer Res. 1972;32(3):583–9.
17. Orth G, Jablonska S, Favre M, Croissant O, Jarzabek-Chorzelska M, Rzesa G. Characterization of two types of human papillomaviruses in lesions of epidermodysplasia verruciformis. Proc Natl Acad Sci U S A. 1978;75(3):1537–41.
18. Orth G, Jablonska S, Jarzabek-Chorzelska M, Obalek S, Rzesa G, Favre M, et al. Characteristics of the lesions and risk of malignant conversion associated with the type of human papillomavirus involved in epidermodysplasia verruciformis. Cancer Res. 1979;39(3):1074–82.
19. Lutzner MA. Epidermodysplasia verruciformis. An autosomal recessive disease characterized by viral warts and skin cancer. A model for viral oncogenesis. Bull Cancer. 1978;65(2):169–82.
20. IARC Working Group on the Evaluation of Carcinogenic Risks to Humans. Human papillomaviruses. IARC Monogr Eval Carcinog Risks Hum. 2007;90:1–636.
21. Bouwes Bavinck JN, Euvrard S, Naldi L, Nindl I, Proby CM, Neale R, et al. Keratotic skin lesions and other risk factors are associated with skin cancer in organ-transplant recipients: a case–control study in The Netherlands, United Kingdom, Germany, France, and Italy. J Invest Dermatol. 2007;127(7):1647–56.
22. Bernard HU, Burk RD, Chen Z, Van DK, zur Hausen H, de Villiers EM. Classification of papillomaviruses (PVs) based on 189 PV types and proposal of taxonomic amendments. Virology. 2010;401(1):70–9.
23. Burk RD, Chen Z, Van DK. Human papillomaviruses: genetic basis of carcinogenicity. Public Health Genomics. 2009;12(5–6):281–90.
24. Zheng ZM, Baker CC. Papillomavirus genome structure, expression, and post-transcriptional regulation. Front Biosci. 2006;11:2286–302.
25. Antonsson A, Forslund O, Ekberg H, Sterner G, Hansson BG. The ubiquity and impressive genomic diversity of human skin papillomaviruses suggest a commensalic nature of these viruses. J Virol. 2000;74(24):11636–41.
26. Boxman IL, Berkhout RJ, Mulder LH, Wolkers MC, Bouwes Bavinck JN, Vermeer BJ, et al. Detection of human papillomavirus DNA in plucked hairs from renal transplant recipients and healthy volunteers. J Invest Dermatol. 1997;108(5):712–5.
27. Feltkamp MC, de Koning MN, Bavinck JN, Ter SJ. Betapapillomaviruses: innocent bystanders or causes of skin cancer. J Clin Virol. 2008;43(4):353–60.
28. Kohler A, Forschner T, Meyer T, Ulrich C, Gottschling M, Stockfleth E, et al. Multifocal distribution of cutaneous human papillomavirus types in hairs from different skin areas. Br J Dermatol. 2007;156(5):1078–80.
29. Weissenborn SJ, de Koning MN, Wieland U, Quint WG, Pfister HJ. Intrafamilial transmission and family-specific spectra of cutaneous betapapillomaviruses. J Virol. 2009;83(2):811–6.
30. Middleton K, Peh W, Southern S, Griffin H, Sotlar K, Nakahara T, et al. Organization of human papillomavirus productive cycle during neoplastic progression provides a basis for selection of diagnostic markers. J Virol. 2003;77(19):10186–201.
31. Peh WL, Middleton K, Christensen N, Nicholls P, Egawa K, Sotlar K, et al. Life cycle heterogeneity in animal models of human papillomavirus-associated disease. J Virol. 2002;76(20):10401–16.
32. Doorbar J. Papillomavirus life cycle organization and biomarker selection. Dis Markers. 2007;23(4):297–313.
33. Egawa K, Iftner A, Doorbar J, Honda Y, Iftner T. Synthesis of viral DNA and late capsid protein L1 in parabasal spinous cell layers of naturally occurring benign warts infected with human papillomavirus type 1. Virology. 2000;268(2):281–93.
34. Aldabagh B, Angeles JG, Cardones AR, Arron ST. Cutaneous squamous cell carcinoma and human papillomavirus: is there an association? Dermatol Surg. 2013;39(1 Pt 1):1–23.
35. Berkhout RJ, Tieben LM, Smits HL, Bavinck JN, Vermeer BJ, Ter SJ. Nested PCR approach for detection and typing of epidermodysplasia verruciformis-associated human papillomavirus types in cutaneous cancers from renal transplant recipients. J Clin Microbiol. 1995;33(3):690–5.
36. Boxman IL, Russell A, Mulder LH, Bavinck JN, ter Schegget JT, Green A. Case–control study in a subtropical Australian population to assess the relation between non-melanoma skin cancer and epidermodysplasia verruciformis human papillomavirus DNA in plucked eyebrow hairs. The Nambour Skin Cancer Prevention Study Group. Int J Cancer. 2000;86(1):118–21.
37. de Jong-Tieben LM, Berkhout RJ, Smits HL, Bouwes Bavinck JN, Vermeer BJ, van der Woude FJ, et al. High frequency of detection of epidermodysplasia verruciformis-associated human papillomavirus DNA in biopsies from malignant and premalignant skin lesions from renal transplant recipients. J Invest Dermatol. 1995;105(3):367–71.
38. de Villiers EM, Lavergne D, McLaren K, Benton EC. Prevailing papillomavirus types in non-melanoma carcinomas of the skin in renal allograft recipients. Int J Cancer. 1997;73(3):356–61.
39. de Koning MN, Quint W, Struijk L, Kleter B, Wanningen P, van Doorn LJ, et al. Evaluation of a novel highly sensitive, broad-spectrum PCR-reverse hybridization assay for detection and identification of beta-papillomavirus DNA. J Clin Microbiol. 2006;44(5):1792–800.
40. Forslund O, Ly H, Higgins G. Improved detection of cutaneous human papillomavirus DNA by single tube nested 'hanging droplet' PCR. J Virol Methods. 2003;110(2):129–36.
41. Gheit T, Billoud G, de Koning MN, Gemignani F, Forslund O, Sylla BS, et al. Development of a sensitive and specific multiplex PCR method combined with DNA microarray primer extension to detect betapapillomavirus types. J Clin Microbiol. 2007;45(8):2537–44.

42. Harwood CA, Spink PJ, Surentheran T, Leigh IM, Hawke JL, Proby CM, et al. Detection of human papillomavirus DNA in PUVA-associated non-melanoma skin cancers. J Invest Dermatol. 1998;111(1):123–7.
43. Nindl I, Koehler A, Meyer T, Forschner T, Meijer CJ, Snijders PJ, et al. Detection of human papillomavirus DNA in primary squamous cell carcinoma and metastases. Br J Dermatol. 2006;154(4):797–9.
44. Weissenborn SJ, Wieland U, Junk M, Pfister H. Quantification of beta-human papillomavirus DNA by real-time PCR. Nat Protoc. 2010;5(1):1–13.
45. Michael KM, Forslund O, Bacevskij O, Waterboer T, Bravo IG, Pawlita M, et al. Bead-based multiplex genotyping of 58 cutaneous human papillomavirus types. J Clin Microbiol. 2011;49(10):3560–7.
46. de Koning MN, Weissenborn SJ, Abeni D, Bouwes Bavinck JN, Euvrard S, Green AC, et al. Prevalence and associated factors of betapapillomavirus infections in individuals without cutaneous squamous cell carcinoma. J Gen Virol. 2009;90(Pt 7):1611–21.
47. Nindl I, Kohler A, Gottschling M, Forschner T, Lehmann M, Meijer CJ, et al. Extension of the typing in a general-primer-PCR reverse-line-blotting system to detect all 25 cutaneous beta human papillomaviruses. J Virol Methods. 2007;146(1–2):1–4.
48. Feltkamp MC, Broer R, di Summa FM, Struijk L, van der Meijden E, Verlaan BP, et al. Seroreactivity to epidermodysplasia verruciformis-related human papillomavirus types is associated with nonmelanoma skin cancer. Cancer Res. 2003;63(10):2695–700.
49. Struijk L, Hall L, van der Meijden E, Wanningen P, Bavinck JN, Neale R, et al. Markers of cutaneous human papillomavirus infection in individuals with tumor-free skin, actinic keratoses, and squamous cell carcinoma. Cancer Epidemiol Biomarkers Prev. 2006;15(3):529–35.
50. Karagas MR, Nelson HH, Sehr P, Waterboer T, Stukel TA, Andrew A, et al. Human papillomavirus infection and incidence of squamous cell and basal cell carcinomas of the skin. J Natl Cancer Inst. 2006;98(6):389–95.
51. Waterboer T, Sehr P, Michael KM, Franceschi S, Nieland JD, Joos TO, et al. Multiplex human papillomavirus serology based on in situ-purified glutathione s-transferase fusion proteins. Clin Chem. 2005;51(10):1845–53.
52. Iftner T, Villa LL. Chapter 12: human papillomavirus technologies. J Natl Cancer Inst Monogr. 2003;31:80–8.
53. Peh WL, Doorbar J. Detection of papillomavirus proteins and DNA in paraffin-embedded tissue sections. Methods Mol Med. 2005;119:49–59.
54. Chew K, Rooney PH, Cruickshank ME, Murray GI. Laser capture microdissection and PCR for analysis of human papilloma virus infection. Methods Mol Biol. 2005;293:295–300.
55. Doorbar J. The papillomavirus life cycle. J Clin Virol. 2005;32 Suppl 1:S7–S15.
56. Longworth MS, Laimins LA. Pathogenesis of human papillomaviruses in differentiating epithelia. Microbiol Mol Biol Rev. 2004;68(2):362–72.
57. Haller K, Stubenrauch F, Pfister H. Differentiation-dependent transcription of the epidermodysplasia verruciformis-associated human papillomavirus type 5 in benign lesions. Virology. 1995;214(1):245–55.
58. Ostrow RS, Bender M, Niimura M, Seki T, Kawashima M, Pass F, et al. Human papillomavirus DNA in cutaneous primary and metastasized squamous cell carcinomas from patients with epidermodysplasia verruciformis. Proc Natl Acad Sci U S A. 1982;79(5):1634–8.
59. Lippens S, Denecker G, Ovaere P, Vandenabeele P, Declercq W. Death penalty for keratinocytes: apoptosis versus cornification. Cell Death Differ. 2005;12 Suppl 2:1497–508.
60. Blanpain C, Fuchs E. Epidermal stem cells of the skin. Annu Rev Cell Dev Biol. 2006;22:339–73.
61. Munger K, Basile JR, Duensing S, Eichten A, Gonzalez SL, Grace M, et al. Biological activities and molecular targets of the human papillomavirus E7 oncoprotein. Oncogene. 2001;20(54):7888–98.
62. zur Hausen H. Immortalization of human cells and their malignant conversion by high risk human papillomavirus genotypes. Semin Cancer Biol. 1999;9(6):405–11.
63. Caldeira S, Zehbe I, Accardi R, Malanchi I, Dong W, Giarre M, et al. The E6 and E7 proteins of the cutaneous human papillomavirus type 38 display transforming properties. J Virol. 2003;77(3):2195–206.
64. Dong WL, Caldeira S, Sehr P, Pawlita M, Tommasino M. Determination of the binding affinity of different human papillomavirus E7 proteins for the tumour suppressor pRb by a plate-binding assay. J Virol Methods. 2001;98(1):91–8.
65. Bedard KM, Underbrink MP, Howie HL, Galloway DA. The E6 oncoproteins from human betapapillomaviruses differentially activate telomerase through an E6AP-dependent mechanism and prolong the lifespan of primary keratinocytes. J Virol. 2008;82(8):3894–902.
66. Cordano P, Gillan V, Bratlie S, Bouvard V, Banks L, Tommasino M, et al. The E6E7 oncoproteins of cutaneous human papillomavirus type 38 interfere with the interferon pathway. Virology. 2008;377(2):408–18.
67. Gabet AS, Accardi R, Bellopede A, Popp S, Boukamp P, Sylla BS, et al. Impairment of the telomere/telomerase system and genomic instability are associated with keratinocyte immortalization induced by the skin human papillomavirus type 38. FASEB J. 2008;22(2):622–32.
68. Accardi R, Dong W, Smet A, Cui R, Hautefeuille A, Gabet AS, et al. Skin human papillomavirus type 38 alters p53 functions by accumulation of deltaNp73. EMBO Rep. 2006;7(3):334–40.
69. Dong W, Arpin C, Accardi R, Gissmann L, Sylla BS, Marvel J, et al. Loss of p53 or p73 in human papillomavirus type 38 E6 and E7 transgenic mice partially restores the UV-activated cell cycle checkpoints. Oncogene. 2008;27(20):2923–8.
70. Akgul B, Garcia-Escudero R, Ghali L, Pfister HJ, Fuchs PG, Navsaria H, et al. The E7 protein of cuta-

neous human papillomavirus type 8 causes invasion of human keratinocytes into the dermis in organotypic cultures of skin. Cancer Res. 2005;65(6):2216–23.
71. Boxman IL, Mulder LH, Noya F, de Waard V, Gibbs S, Broker TR, et al. Transduction of the E6 and E7 genes of epidermodysplasia-verruciformis-associated human papillomaviruses alters human keratinocyte growth and differentiation in organotypic cultures. J Invest Dermatol. 2001;117(6):1397–404.
72. Kazem S, van der Meijden E, Struijk L, de Gruijl FR, Feltkamp MC. Human papillomavirus 8 E6 disrupts terminal skin differentiation and prevents pro-Caspase-14 cleavage. Virus Res. 2012;163(2):609–16.
73. Bouwes Bavinck JN, Feltkamp MC. Milk of human kindness?–HAMLET, human papillomavirus, and warts. N Engl J Med. 2004;350(26):2639–42.
74. Jackson S, Harwood C, Thomas M, Banks L, Storey A. Role of Bak in UV-induced apoptosis in skin cancer and abrogation by HPV E6 proteins. Genes Dev. 2000;14(23):3065–73.
75. Jackson S, Storey A. E6 proteins from diverse cutaneous HPV types inhibit apoptosis in response to UV damage. Oncogene. 2000;19(4):592–8.
76. Leverrier S, Bergamaschi D, Ghali L, Ola A, Warnes G, Akgul B, et al. Role of HPV E6 proteins in preventing UVB-induced release of pro-apoptotic factors from the mitochondria. Apoptosis. 2007;12(3):549–60.
77. Struijk L, van der Meijden E, Kazem S, Ter SJ, de Gruijl FR, Steenbergen RD, et al. Specific betapapillomaviruses associated with squamous cell carcinoma of the skin inhibit UVB-induced apoptosis of primary human keratinocytes. J Gen Virol. 2008;89(Pt 9):2303–14.
78. Underbrink MP, Howie HL, Bedard KM, Koop JI, Galloway DA. E6 proteins from multiple human betapapillomavirus types degrade Bak and protect keratinocytes from apoptosis after UVB irradiation. J Virol. 2008;82(21):10408–17.
79. Pfister H. Chapter 8: human papillomavirus and skin cancer. J Natl Cancer Inst Monogr. 2003;31:52–6.
80. Viarisio D, Mueller-Decker K, Kloz U, Aengeneyndt B, Kopp-Schneider A, Grone HJ, et al. E6 and E7 from beta HPV38 cooperate with ultraviolet light in the development of actinic keratosis-like lesions and squamous cell carcinoma in mice. PLoS Pathog. 2011;7(7):e1002125.
81. Hall L, Struijk L, Neale RE, Feltkamp MC. Re: human papillomavirus infection and incidence of squamous cell and basal cell carcinomas of the skin. J Natl Cancer Inst. 2006;98(19):1425–6.
82. Mendoza JA, Jacob Y, Cassonnet P, Favre M. Human papillomavirus type 5 E6 oncoprotein represses the transforming growth factor beta signaling pathway by binding to SMAD3. J Virol. 2006;80(24):12420–4.
83. Rozenblatt-Rosen O, Deo RC, Padi M, Adelmant G, Calderwood MA, Rolland T, et al. Interpreting cancer genomes using systematic host network perturbations by tumour virus proteins. Nature. 2012;487(7408):491–5.
84. Weissenborn SJ, Nindl I, Purdie K, Harwood C, Proby C, Breuer J, et al. Human papillomavirus-DNA loads in actinic keratoses exceed those in non-melanoma skin cancers. J Invest Dermatol. 2005;125(1):93–7.
85. Andersson K, Waterboer T, Kirnbauer R, Slupetzky K, Iftner T, de Villiers EM, et al. Seroreactivity to cutaneous human papillomaviruses among patients with nonmelanoma skin cancer or benign skin lesions. Cancer Epidemiol Biomarkers Prev. 2008;17(1):189–95.
86. Antonsson A, Karanfilovska S, Lindqvist PG, Hansson BG. General acquisition of human papillomavirus infections of skin occurs in early infancy. J Clin Microbiol. 2003;41(6):2509–14.
87. Bouwes Bavinck JN, Neale RE, Abeni D, Euvrard S, Green AC, Harwood CA, et al. Multicenter study of the association between betapapillomavirus infection and cutaneous squamous cell carcinoma. Cancer Res. 2010;70(23):9777–86.
88. Boxman IL, Mulder LH, Russell A, Bouwes Bavinck JN, Green A, Ter SJ. Human papillomavirus type 5 is commonly present in immunosuppressed and immunocompetent individuals. Br J Dermatol. 1999;141(2):246–9.
89. de Koning MN, Struijk L, Bavinck JN, Kleter B, Ter SJ, Quint WG, et al. Betapapillomaviruses frequently persist in the skin of healthy individuals. J Gen Virol. 2007;88(Pt 5):1489–95.
90. Hsu JY, Chen AC, Keleher A, McMillan NA, Antonsson A. Shared and persistent asymptomatic cutaneous human papillomavirus infections in healthy skin. J Med Virol. 2009;81(8):1444–9.
91. Alotaibi L, Provost N, Gagnon S, Franco EL, Coutlee F. Diversity of cutaneous human papillomavirus types in individuals with and without skin lesion. J Clin Virol. 2006;36(2):133–40.
92. Antonsson A, Erfurt C, Hazard K, Holmgren V, Simon M, Kataoka A, et al. Prevalence and type spectrum of human papillomaviruses in healthy skin samples collected in three continents. J Gen Virol. 2003;84(Pt 7):1881–6.
93. Forslund O, Antonsson A, Nordin P, Stenquist B, Hansson BG. A broad range of human papillomavirus types detected with a general PCR method suitable for analysis of cutaneous tumours and normal skin. J Gen Virol. 1999;80(Pt 9):2437–43.
94. Forslund O, Ly H, Reid C, Higgins G. A broad spectrum of human papillomavirus types is present in the skin of Australian patients with non-melanoma skin cancers and solar keratosis. Br J Dermatol. 2003;149(1):64–73.
95. Hazard K, Karlsson A, Andersson K, Ekberg H, Dillner J, Forslund O. Cutaneous human papillomaviruses persist on healthy skin. J Invest Dermatol. 2007;127(1):116–9.
96. Chen AC, McMillan NA, Antonsson A. Human papillomavirus type spectrum in normal skin of individuals with or without a history of frequent sun exposure. J Gen Virol. 2008;89(Pt 11):2891–7.
97. Iannacone MR, Michael KM, Giuliano AR, Waterboer T, Pawlita M, Rollison DE. Risk factors for cutaneous human papillomavirus seroreactivity among patients undergoing skin cancer screening in Florida. J Infect Dis. 2010;201(5):760–9.

98. Waterboer T, Neale R, Michael KM, Sehr P, de Koning MN, Weissenborn SJ, et al. Antibody responses to 26 skin human papillomavirus types in the Netherlands, Italy and Australia. J Gen Virol. 2009;90(Pt 8):1986–98.
99. Michael KM, Waterboer T, Sehr P, Rother A, Reidel U, Boeing H, et al. Seroprevalence of 34 human papillomavirus types in the German general population. PLoS Pathog. 2008;4(6):e1000091.
100. Antonsson A, Waterboer T, Bouwes Bavinck JN, Abeni D, de Koning M, Euvrard S, et al. Longitudinal study of seroprevalence and serostability of 34 human papillomavirus types in European organ transplant recipients. Virology. 2013;436(1):91–9.
101. Casabonne D, Waterboer T, Michael KM, Pawlita M, Lally A, Mitchell L, et al. The sero-epidemiology of human papillomavirus among Caucasian transplant recipients in the UK. Infect Agent Cancer. 2009;4:13.
102. Asgari MM, Kiviat NB, Critchlow CW, Stern JE, Argenyi ZB, Raugi GJ, et al. Detection of human papillomavirus DNA in cutaneous squamous cell carcinoma among immunocompetent individuals. J Invest Dermatol. 2008;128(6):1409–17.
103. Forslund O, Iftner T, Andersson K, Lindelof B, Hradil E, Nordin P, et al. Cutaneous human papillomaviruses found in sun-exposed skin: beta-papillomavirus species 2 predominates in squamous cell carcinoma. J Infect Dis. 2007;196(6):876–83.
104. Meyer T, Arndt R, Christophers E, Nindl I, Stockfleth E. Importance of human papillomaviruses for the development of skin cancer. Cancer Detect Prev. 2001;25(6):533–47.
105. Patel AS, Karagas MR, Perry AE, Nelson HH. Exposure profiles and human papillomavirus infection in skin cancer: an analysis of 25 genus beta-types in a population-based study. J Invest Dermatol. 2008;128(12):2888–93.
106. Pfister H, Fuchs PG, Majewski S, Jablonska S, Pniewska I, Malejczyk M. High prevalence of epidermodysplasia verruciformis-associated human papillomavirus DNA in actinic keratoses of the immunocompetent population. Arch Dermatol Res. 2003;295(7):273–9.
107. Plasmeijer EI, Neale RE, Buettner PG, de Koning MN, ter Schegget J, Quint WG, et al. Betapapillomavirus infection profiles in tissue sets from cutaneous squamous cell-carcinoma patients. Int J Cancer. 2010;126(11):2614–21.
108. Berkhout RJ, Bouwes Bavinck JN, Ter SJ. Persistence of human papillomavirus DNA in benign and (pre) malignant skin lesions from renal transplant recipients. J Clin Microbiol. 2000;38(6):2087–96.
109. Meyer T, Arndt R, Nindl I, Ulrich C, Christophers E, Stockfleth E. Association of human papillomavirus infections with cutaneous tumors in immunosuppressed patients. Transpl Int. 2003;16(3):146–53.
110. de Jong-Tieben LM, Berkhout RJ, Ter SJ, Vermeer BJ, de Fijter JW, Bruijn JA, et al. The prevalence of human papillomavirus DNA in benign keratotic skin lesions of renal transplant recipients with and without a history of skin cancer is equally high: a clinical study to assess risk factors for keratotic skin lesions and skin cancer. Transplantation. 2000;69(1):44–9.
111. Mackintosh LJ, de Koning MN, Quint WG, Ter SJ, Morgan IM, Herd RM, et al. Presence of beta human papillomaviruses in nonmelanoma skin cancer from organ transplant recipients and immunocompetent patients in the West of Scotland. Br J Dermatol. 2009;161(1):56–62.
112. Boxman IL, Russell A, Mulder LH, Bavinck JN, Ter SJ, Green A. Association between epidermodysplasia verruciformis-associated human papillomavirus DNA in plucked eyebrow hair and solar keratoses. J Invest Dermatol. 2001;117(5):1108–12.
113. Struijk L, Bouwes Bavinck JN, Wanningen P, van der Meijden E, Westendorp RG, Ter SJ, et al. Presence of human papillomavirus DNA in plucked eyebrow hairs is associated with a history of cutaneous squamous cell carcinoma. J Invest Dermatol. 2003;121(6):1531–5.
114. Harwood CA, Surentheran T, Sasieni P, Proby CM, Bordea C, Leigh IM, et al. Increased risk of skin cancer associated with the presence of epidermodysplasia verruciformis human papillomavirus types in normal skin. Br J Dermatol. 2004;150(5):949–57.
115. McBride P, Neale R, Pandeya N, Green A. Sun-related factors, betapapillomavirus, and actinic keratoses: a prospective study. Arch Dermatol. 2007;143(7):862–8.
116. Proby CM, Harwood CA, Neale RE, Green AC, Euvrard S, Naldi L, et al. A case–control study of betapapillomavirus infection and cutaneous squamous cell carcinoma in organ transplant recipients. Am J Transplant. 2011;11(7):1498–508.
117. Neale RE, Weissenborn S, Abeni D, Bavinck JN, Euvrard S, Feltkamp MC, et al. Human papillomavirus load in eyebrow hair follicles and risk of cutaneous squamous cell carcinoma. Cancer Epidemiol Biomarkers Prev. 2013;22(4):719–27.
118. Bzhalava D, Guan P, Franceschi S, Dillner J, Clifford G. A systematic review of the prevalence of mucosal and cutaneous human papillomavirus types. Virology. 2013;445(1–2):224–31.
119. Steger G, Olszewsky M, Stockfleth E, Pfister H. Prevalence of antibodies to human papillomavirus type 8 in human sera. J Virol. 1990;64(9):4399–406.
120. Stark S, Petridis AK, Ghim SJ, Jenson AB, Bouwes Bavinck JN, Gross G, et al. Prevalence of antibodies against virus-like particles of epidermodysplasia verruciformis-associated HPV8 in patients at risk of skin cancer. J Invest Dermatol. 1998;111(4):696–701.
121. Bouwes Bavinck JN, Stark S, Petridis AK, Marugg ME, Ter SJ, Westendorp RG, et al. The presence of antibodies against virus-like particles of epidermodysplasia verruciformis-associated human papillomavirus type 8 in patients with actinic keratoses. Br J Dermatol. 2000;142(1):103–9.
122. Masini C, Fuchs PG, Gabrielli F, Stark S, Sera F, Ploner M, et al. Evidence for the association of human papillomavirus infection and cutaneous squa-

mous cell carcinoma in immunocompetent individuals. Arch Dermatol. 2003;139(7):890–4.
123. Casabonne D, Waterboer T, Michael KM, Pawlita M, Mitchell L, Newton R, et al. The seroprevalence of human papillomavirus by immune status and by ethnicity in London. Infect Agent Cancer. 2009;4:14.
124. Karagas MR, Waterboer T, Li Z, Nelson HH, Michael KM, Bavinck JN, et al. Genus beta human papillomaviruses and incidence of basal cell and squamous cell carcinomas of skin: population based case–control study. BMJ. 2010;341:c2986.
125. Waterboer T, Abeni D, Sampogna F, Rother A, Masini C, Sehr P, et al. Serological association of beta and gamma human papillomaviruses with squamous cell carcinoma of the skin. Br J Dermatol. 2008;159(2):457–9.
126. Plasmeijer EI, Pandeya N, O'Rourke P, Pawlita M, Waterboer T, Feltkamp MC, et al. The association between cutaneous squamous cell carcinoma and betapapillomavirus seropositivity: a cohort study. Cancer Epidemiol Biomarkers Prev. 2011;20(6):1171–7.
127. Paradisi A, Waterboer T, Sampogna F, Tabolli S, Simoni S, Pawlita M, et al. Seropositivity for human papillomavirus and incidence of subsequent squamous cell and basal cell carcinomas of the skin in patients with a previous nonmelanoma skin cancer. Br J Dermatol. 2011;165(4):782–91.
128. Casabonne D, Michael KM, Waterboer T, Pawlita M, Forslund O, Burk RD, et al. A prospective pilot study of antibodies against human papillomaviruses and cutaneous squamous cell carcinoma nested in the Oxford component of the European Prospective Investigation into Cancer and Nutrition. Int J Cancer. 2007;121(8):1862–8.
129. Purdie KJ, Surentheran T, Sterling JC, Bell L, McGregor JM, Proby CM, et al. Human papillomavirus gene expression in cutaneous squamous cell carcinomas from immunosuppressed and immunocompetent individuals. J Invest Dermatol. 2005;125(1):98–107.
130. Dang C, Koehler A, Forschner T, Sehr P, Michael K, Pawlita M, et al. E6/E7 expression of human papillomavirus types in cutaneous squamous cell dysplasia and carcinoma in immunosuppressed organ transplant recipients. Br J Dermatol. 2006;155(1):129–36.
131. Arron ST, Ruby JG, Dybbro E, Ganem D, Derisi JL. Transcriptome sequencing demonstrates that human papillomavirus is not active in cutaneous squamous cell carcinoma. J Invest Dermatol. 2011;131(8):1745–53.
132. Iannacone MR, Gheit T, Waterboer T, Giuliano AR, Messina JL, Fenske NA, et al. Case–control study of cutaneous human papillomavirus infection in Basal cell carcinoma of the skin. J Invest Dermatol. 2013;133(6):1512–20.
133. Paolini F, Carbone A, Benevolo M, Silipo V, Rollo F, Covello R, et al. Human papillomaviruses, p16INK4a and Akt expression in basal cell carcinoma. J Exp Clin Cancer Res. 2011;30:108.

4 Advances in Our Understanding of Immunosuppression as a Risk Factor for Cutaneous SCC: Evidence for Revision of Immunosuppressive Therapy

Günther F.L. Hofbauer and Chantal C. Bachmann

Contents

G.F.L. Hofbauer, MD (✉) • C.C. Bachmann, MD
Dermatologische Klinik, UniversitätsSpital Zürich, Gloriastrasse 31, Zürich 8091, Switzerland
e-mail: hofbauer@usz.ch; chantal.bachmann@usz.ch

Abbreviations

AZA	Azathioprine
BCC	Basal cell carcinoma
CNI	Calcineurin inhibitors such as cyclosporine A tacrolimus
CsA	Cyclosporine A
HPV	Human papillomavirus
MM	Melanoma
MMF	Mycophenolate mofetil
NHL	Non-Hodgkin lymphoma
NMSC	Nonmelanoma skin cancer
OTR	Organ transplant recipient
P	Prednisolone steroids
SCC	Squamous cell carcinoma
TAC	Tacrolimus

4.1 Introduction

Organ transplant recipients (OTRs) on immunosuppressive therapy are at increased risk of nonmelanoma skin cancer (NMSC) including epithelial skin cancer, Merkel cell carcinoma, and Kaposi's sarcoma, as well as other transplant-associated cancers compared to the normal population [1]. Squamous cell carcinoma (SCC) of the skin is a major complication of treatment with immunosuppressive drugs, with a 65- to 100-fold higher risk than in the normal population [2]. Other malignancies like basal cell carcinoma (BCC), melanoma, and internal malignancies increase as well but to a significantly lesser extent [3].

F. Zwald, M.D. Brown (eds.), *Advances in Transplant Dermatology: Clinical and Practical Implications*,
DOI 10.1007/978-3-319-12445-2_4, © Springer International Publishing Switzerland 2015

The incidence of SCC depends on the grafted organ, UV light exposure, genetic factors, immunological control of oncogenic viruses, and the dose, intensity, and duration of the immunosuppressive drug [1, 4–6]. These contributing factors are discussed in earlier chapters (e.g., 2 and 3). Patients suffering of lymphoma or leukemia as well patients on biologic therapies have a higher risk to develop SCC and are more likely to die of SCC metastasis [7]. While the individual impact of each immunosuppressant on carcinogenesis in clinical practice has eluded us to date, we have increased our understanding of immunosuppressants and carcinogenesis of the skin over the last decade and will address these advances below.

4.2 Total Immunosuppression and Carcinogenesis

Suppression of the immune system leads to an increased risk in cancer. While several drivers coincide in the formation of skin cancer following transplantation, the immunosuppressive role plays a central role and contributes greatly to cutaneous carcinogenesis in OTR [2, 8]. The incidence of skin cancer is related to the depth and length of immunosuppression in general [2].

Following transplantation, the incidence of skin cancer increases over time. BCC seems to develop after transplantation with a linear relative risk (annual incidence of 0.173 %) and SCC even exponentially ($r'=0.739$) [4, 9, 10]. SCC is observed more rapidly and more frequently after transplantation in OTR older at transplantation. OTR above 60 years of age showed a median time to the first SCC after transplantation of 3 years, while those aged 18–40 years at time of transplantation showed a median delay of 13 years to their first SCC ($P>0.001$) [9].

Pronounced immunosuppression seems to be one reason for an increased risk for NMSC. Heart transplant recipients with poor graft function in the first year with multiple rejection episodes and consecutively higher cumulative immunosuppression load showed a higher risk of skin cancer [11]. Various studies, for example, Euvrard et al. [12] and Jensen et al. [13], reported a higher risk for SCC growth in OTR with profound immunosuppression after heart transplantation compared to lower levels which are used in liver or kidney transplant recipients. Jensen et al. [13] compared the outcome for NMSC incidence between triple and double immunosuppressive therapy in kidney and heart transplant recipients. The risk of developing SCC was 4.2 times higher (95 % confidence interval, 2.1–8.5) in the group receiving triple immunosuppressants compared to the group receiving only double immunosuppressive therapy with azathioprine and prednisolone. Another study of Euvrard et al. demonstrated already in 1995 that the incidence for skin cancer was twice as high for heart transplant recipients compared to kidney transplant recipients. It was presumed to be due to higher doses of immunosuppression in the heart transplant group [14]. In 2006, Euvrard investigated the risk for subsequent skin cancers after the first NMSC in OTRs. Heart transplant recipients developed proportionally more skin cancer than kidney transplant recipients, but the mean number was lower for the heart transplant recipients. An explanation could be that kidney transplant patients are at a younger age at the time of transplantation and therefore receive a longer period of immunosuppression [62].

It remains difficult to gauge the actual impact of total immunosuppression on skin cancer formation. It has been found that a decreased CD4 cell count associates with the subsequent development of skin cancers in patients after kidney transplantation. Is seems possible that NMSC formation is specifically related to CD4 depletion because there was no visible relationship between skin cancer and CD8, CD19, and lymphopenia in general [15].

It is still uncertain if the drug class, dose, or combinations are the most important for NMSC formation [2]. A multidrug regimen is the rule in immunosuppression to prevent rejection. While these regimes are frequently similar, they are not identical and vary in composition and over time. No study has therefore been able to isolate the effect of individual compounds yet. We know that NMSC risk increases with the number of immunosuppressive agents: One study assessed skin cancer incidence in OTR on long-term monotherapy with a calcineurin inhibitor compared to bi- or tri-therapy among the first renal allograft recipients 6 years or longer after transplantation. The groups were not identical, as monotherapy was more frequent in older OTR who had longer follow-up and had suffered fewer biopsy-proven acute rejection episodes. Not only was a higher graft survival rate observed in the monotherapy group, but there was also a clear reduction in skin cancer incidence after 12 years post-transplantation. Abou Ayache concludes that calcineurin monotherapy in selected patients can be considered as a minimization strategy for immunosuppression against SCC formation [16].

Compared to patients on bi-therapy with azathioprine and corticosteroids, OTR on a triple immunosuppressive therapy with cyclosporine A (CsA), azathioprine (AZA), and corticosteroids (prednisolone, P) was found to have a three times elevated risk of skin cancer [2, 13, 17]. One recent study dissected different immunosuppressive regimes for their association with skin cancer. The combination of CsA, AZA, and P associated with tumors in 5.2 % of patients. The combination of mycophenolate mofetil (MMF) with CsA and P associated with tumors in 3.4 % of OTR, whereas MMF, P, and tacrolimus (TAC) associated with tumors in 3.3 % of OTR, and AZA and P with 10 %, respectively. Paired comparison ranked the combination of AZA with P the highest for risk of malignancy, of note; however, these OTRs also had been followed up the longest. CsA and AZA combined with P stood out compared to the combinations of CsA, MMF, and P or TAC, MMF, and P. OTR on TAC+MMF+P showed an earlier onset of tumors. The tumor-free survival was shortest for AZA+P and longest for the combination of MMF and TAC with P ($p<0.001$) [18]. To learn more about the impact of total immunosuppression and the respective contributing drugs, it will take further structured cohort studies to collect data on immunosuppressive agents and skin cancer formation (Fig. 4.1).

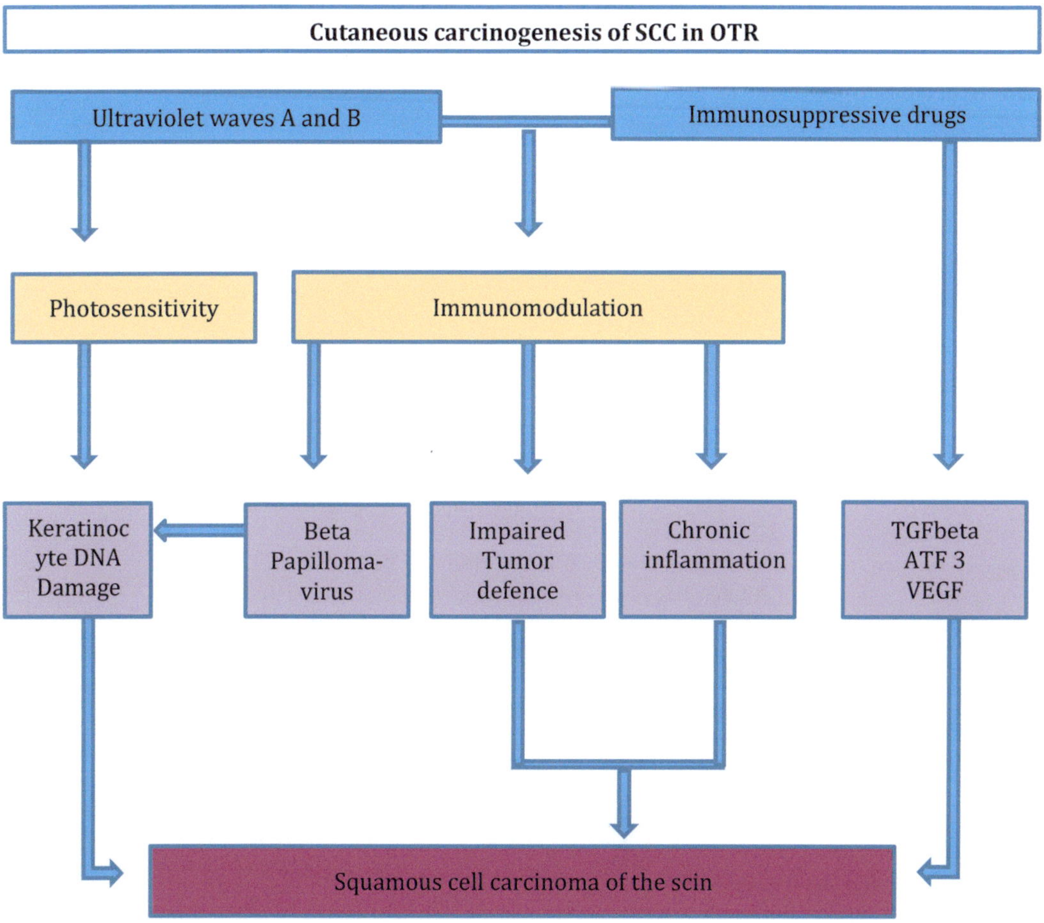

Fig. 4.1 Cutaneous carcinogenesis of SCC in OTR

4.3 Effects of Individual Immunosuppressive Drugs (Table 4.1)

4.3.1 Glucocorticoids

Several studies have addressed the association of steroid use with cutaneous carcinogenesis. The use of systemic glucocorticoids for more than 1 month in diverse indications other than OTR doubles the risk for squamous cell carcinoma (relative risk for steroid use 2.31 (95 % confidence interval 1.27–4.18)). Oral glucocorticoids increased the risk for SCC in patients other than OTR (adjusted odds ratio = 2.31; 95 % CI = 1.27, 4.18) [20], while the risk of BCC did not change. A Danish study found an increased risk for basal cell carcinoma, squamous cell carcinoma, and non-Hodgkin lymphoma in patients on systemic glucocorticoids longer than a month in non-OTR patients [21]. Additional studies suggest oral glucocorticoids as a risk factor for slightly increased BCC risk in the general population where the ratio of incidence increased to 1.17 (95 % CI: 1.08–1.28) for use beyond 1 year and to 1.22 (95 % CI: 1.09–1.36) for use beyond 5 years before the development of BCC [22]. On the other hand, inhaled corticosteroids did not have an impact of SCC and BCC formation, probably due to the modest systemic steroid absorption [20].

Until now, a mechanism for glucocorticoids in skin cancer formation has not been defined. It is assumed that glucocorticoids reduce the tumor surveillance by the immune system in multifactorial ways.

4.3.2 Calcineurin Inhibitors

Calcineurin inhibitors (CNIs) such as cyclosporine A (CsA) and the ascomycin-related drugs tacrolimus and pimecrolimus belong to this class. They inhibit calcineurin mainly in lymphocytes, thus impeding the nuclear localization of the transcription factor nuclear factor of activated T cells (NFAT). This blockade represses cytokines and chemokines needed for T-cell activation. The result is a profound systemic suppression of the immune system focused on T lymphocytes (reviewed in Reynolds and Al-Daraji [19]).

In OTR with systemic calcineurin inhibitor therapy, there is an immediate rise in incidence of SCC directly after transplantation without delay. Stopping CNI shows a decrease of the SCC incidence [23]. Compared to standard CsA dose (150–250 ng/m), a low-dose CsA therapy (75–125 ng/mL) shows a decrease of NMSC incidence. In the standard regime, 26 patients out of 115 suffered of NMSC compared with 17 out of 116 patients in the low-dose group. Unfortunately,

Table 4.1 Effects of individual immunosuppressive drugs

Drug	Effect	Literature
Glucocorticoids	Possibly impair tumor surveillance, increase risk for SCC, BCC, and non-Hodgkin lymphoma	[20–22]
Calcineurin inhibitors	Increase the expression of TGF beta, VEGF (increasing angiogenesis and tumor growth), and ATF3 (impacting p53), decreases DNA repair following UV exposure	[23, 24, 26–32, 34]
	Increased risk for SCC	
Azathioprine	Photosensitizes to UVA and increases DNA damage, reduces DNA repair activity	[35–40]
	Increases risk for SCC more than BCC	
Mycophenolate mofetil	Antioxidative activity by inhibition of 2 NAD(p)H oxidase, reduces angiogenesis	[41–44]
	Lower risk for NMSC than other antimetabolites, no risk for lymphoma	
mTOR inhibitors	Inhibit IL-2 signaling, antitumoral and antiangiogenic potential (inhibits VEGF and TGF beta)	[29, 45–61]
	Lower risk for SCC than CNI	

patients with lower CsA therapy demonstrated more transplant rejection episodes as a limiting problem [24]. A single-center cohort study compared the outcome of cancer including skin cancer following renal transplantation from CsA in 798 patients to tacrolimus in 355 patients. The study concluded that there was no difference between two groups regarding skin cancer formation for the use of induction or maintenance therapy [25].

CNI leads to cancer formation by increasing the expression of transforming growth factor beta (TGF beta) [26]. A dose dependency was seen for tacrolimus on tumor growth and TGF-beta1 cytokine expression in mice, where this overexpression by tacrolimus provides immunosuppressive signals and contributes to tumor progression [27]. Compared to CsA, tacrolimus is associated with a minor increase of the TGF-b transcription rate in humans [28]. CsA also induces the expression of vascular endothelial growth factor (VEGF) [29]. Neoangiogenesis driven by VEGF probably drives tumor growth and metastasis. While general immunosuppression by CNI is certainly driving skin cancer formation, CNI also directly affects keratinocytes and thus contributes to cancer formation of the skin in particular. Several mechanisms have been delineated as contributors to the clearly recognizable increase in tumor formation for patients on these compounds.

DNA repair was shown to be inhibited in lymphocytes from OTR on CsA and ascomycin, lagging behind in compensating for UV-induced damage. The UV-induced apoptosis in human keratinocytes was impaired as well. Both of these phenomena were observed at therapeutic doses of CsA. Apoptosis and necrosis were less visible at low CsA doses of 125 and 250 nM, with a more pronounced effect at 125 nM [30]. The persisting DNA damage is a risk factor for skin cancer formation. Apoptosis protects our cells from cancer formation including skin cancer, whereas the reduction of apoptosis by CsA is an initiating factor for cancer. In summary, CNI increases NMSC formation in two ways: DNA damage and the reduction of apoptotic removal of such cells [31].

CsA shows effects on the mitochondria where it inhibits the opening of mitochondrial permeability transition pore (MPTP). Oxidative stress induced by UV light leads to opening of MPTP, mediating cell death. CsA now promotes survival of damaged cells, allowing for tumor development. The model used showed CsA to prevent cell death in this manner, while TAC had no such effect. CsA rather than TAC may thus drive cutaneous carcinogenesis by prolonged keratinocyte survival following genotoxic stress [30].

Xunwei Wu et al. [32] reported that under CNI, the transcription factor ATF3 is selectively upregulated. ATF3 belongs to the family of AP-1 transcription factors in keratinocytes. ATF3 has a direct impact of tumor formation in keratinocytes by downregulating the mRNA expression of p53 and consecutively the p53-dependent senescence. Recent data demonstrated that UVA light increases ATF3 expression in keratinocytes also in the general population independent of CNI medication. This may be the reason why SCC appears in OTR on CNI preferably on chronically sun-exposed skin [33, 34].

In summary, CNI increases skin cancer formation both by immune-mediated effects such as reduced tumor surveillance by inactivation of lymphocytes and TGF beta secretion, promotes growth and metastasis by VEGF, and directly drives keratinocytes into skin cancer by reduced DNA repair following UV damage, interference with mitochondrial MPTP, and increased ATF3 expression impacting p53 which is potentiated by UVA.

4.3.3 Azathioprine

Azathioprine (AZA) is a purine analog which inhibits purine synthesis and metabolism by incorporation of its metabolite 6-thioguanine into the DNA. OTRs with long-term use of azathioprine have an 8.8-fold increased risk of nonmelanoma skin cancer [35]. Immunosuppressive therapy in organ transplant recipients has a stronger impact on the incidence of squamous cell carcinoma than on basal cell carcinoma [13]. AZA counts as risk factor for developing SCC after a total treatment duration of more than 11 years or a cumulative individual dose of more than 500 g AZA. Patients being on AZA therapy for autoimmune inflammatory rheumatism were recognized to have a significantly increased risk of developing SCC (OR 30 (95 % CI 2.6–345.1) and OR 13.5 (95 % CI 1.3–143.6)) without correcting for risk factors, compared to the general population. After the start of AZA, the time to develop SCC ranged from 3.5 to 15.2 years (median 11.3 years) [36].

AZA not only leads to cancer formation by immunosuppression, it is – not unlike CNI – also directly carcinogenic. AZA increases the oxidative DNA damage caused by UVA irradiation in keratinocytes [37]. UVA damages DNA by radical oxygen species in keratinocytes. AZA converts to its active metabolite 6-thioguanine (6-TG) inserted as base analog into DNA of dividing cells. 6-TG DNA preferentially absorbs UVA and, as a first step in cancer formation, induces DNA strand breaks [37]. Kidney transplant recipients under AZA treatment showed a reduced minimal erythema dose for UVA and an increase in p53 mutant foci, while the DNA repair activity was reduced in human keratinocytes [38]. In hairless albino mice, AZA increases the risk of ultraviolet radiation-induced skin cancer. Thirty weeks after the start of UVA and AZA treatment, the mean number of cancers per mouse was 4.38 ($p<0.05$) [39]. Stopping azathioprine normalizes the photosensitivity to UVA, while this process takes up to 2 years [40].

4.4 Mycophenolate Mofetil

Mycophenolate mofetil (MMF) is the ethyl ester of the fungal antibiotic mycophenolic acid, which inhibits the de novo purine biosynthesis pathway. MMF is currently widely used in replacement of AZA and is part of a typical initial immunosuppressive regimen in kidney transplantation.

Compared with other antimetabolites, MMF was proven to be a lower risk for malignancies in general, including skin cancer [41]. James et al. looked for associations in the development of malignancy [42]. Patients on MMF therapy had a lower incidence of skin cancers compared to patients on AZA (adjusted RR=0.73, 95 % confidence interval 0.25–1.03, $p=0.09$). There was also a slightly lower risk for PTLD/lymphoma in the MMF group (adjusted RR=0.44, 95 % confidence interval 0.19–1.01, $p=0.054$). In total, the adjusted risk for skin cancer formation was reduced on MMF by 27 % (p value 0.02, relative risk 0.73, 95 % confidence limits for relative risk 0.56–0.95) [42]. Another positive finding was the unchanged risk for lymphoma formation on MMF compared to patients receiving other immunosuppressive treatments [43].

MMF is known to reduce angiogenesis and consequently tumor growth. Studies proclaim antioxidant activity for MMF. In contrast to calcineurin inhibitors like CsA, MMF decreases endothelial O_2 formation (superoxide anions) by inhibition of the 2 NAD(P)H oxidase. CsA increased the 2 NAD(P)H oxidase activity resulting in O_2 formation. Endothelial dysfunction is induced by increases in production of reactive oxygen species, such as superoxide anions produced by NAD(P)H oxidase [44].

4.4.1 Mammalian Target of Rapamycin (mTOR) Inhibitors

Inhibitors of the mammalian target of rapamycin (mTOR), including sirolimus and everolimus, are newer immunosuppressants. mTOR participates in key cellular processes such as protein translation, ribosome biosynthesis, and the regulation of the cell cycle. The immune system is influenced by mTOR at the level of lymphocyte proliferation, as well as angiogenesis and wound healing, and the proliferation of cancer cells [45].

In T cells, mTOR inhibitors block IL-2 signaling: sirolimus – a structural analog of the macrolide antibiotic FK 506 – enters into a complex with the intracellular FK-binding protein-12 (FKBP12) which exhibits high affinity to mTOR. mTOR inhibition dephosphorylates and inactivates in turn the p70 ribosomal protein S6 kinase. In consequence, the cell cycle is arrested at the juncture of G1 and S phase. As a result, IL-2 activation of lymphocyte proliferation and immunoglobulin production are impaired [46].

Sirolimus is a potent non-nephrotoxic immunosuppressant which – similar to MMF – has been recognized to reduce the incidence of malignancies in OTRs by its antitumoral and antiangiogenic features [47, 48].

The effect of sirolimus on the growth of various cancer cell lines has been studied in mice. Compared with control mice, sirolimus-treated mice have shown a diminished tumor growth. In sirolimus-treated mice, VEGF secretion and subsequently the circulating levels of VEGF and TGF-beta1 were lower [2, 45].

VEGF is a key mediator of angiogenesis. mTOR inhibition by sirolimus mediates antiangiogenic effects by lowering VEGF and reducing the endothelial response to VEGF. In addition to the antiangiogenic action, sirolimus inhibits proliferation of tumors in mice [29].

There are two separate mTOR-signaling complexes: mTOR complex 1 (mTORC1) and mTOR complex 2 (mTORC2). Sirolimus inhibits the mTOR pathway by directly binding mTORC1, whereas everolimus, a derivative of sirolimus, targets the mTORC1 protein, not the mTORC2 protein. Sirolimus and everolimus share a common structure and mechanism but differ in their serum half-life (60 h for sirolimus and 30 h for everolimus, respectively) [3]. Compared to AZA and CsA, mTOR inhibitors have a protective antitumoral effect including for NMSC in OTRs by controlling signals of the carcinogenic pathway and are still powerful immunosuppressive agents [45].

In comparison to conventional immunosuppressive agents, it is believed that mTOR inhibitors also show antitumoral effects through their influence on immune cells. Six months after switching from CNI and AZA to sirolimus FOXP3$^+$ T cells and NK cells, numbers are increased. It is unclear whether discontinuance of CNI/AZA or the introduction of mTOR inhibitors is responsible for these changes in immune phenotype. Elevation of NK cell levels should act protectively against NMSC formation, but the elevation of FOXP3+ T cell number is believed to carry the risk of later cancer formation. The increase of FOXP3 T-cell levels in OTRs after discontinuance of CNI and/or switching to mTOR inhibitors could be a marker for transplant recipients who are at higher risk of new NMSC formation even with the antitumoral impact of sirolimus [49].

Mathew et al. compared in 1,295 kidney transplant recipients different sirolimus therapy regimes and the outcome after 2 years post transplantation regarding malignancies in general. The first group received sirolimus in continuous combination with CsA, the second, sirolimus as base therapy, and the third, sirolimus maintenance therapy after early withdrawal of CsA. The results of the first group demonstrated that 2 years after transplantation, patients receiving placebo had a higher (6.9 %) incidence of malignancies than OTRs receiving sirolimus in continuous combination with CsA. In the second group, kidney transplant recipients receiving sirolimus as base therapy had no malignancies compared with a 5 % incidence in patients receiving CsA. The malignancy rate in the third group was higher in OTRs receiving sirolimus plus CsA compared to patients on sirolimus therapy with early elimination of CsA (Fig. 4.2) [50].

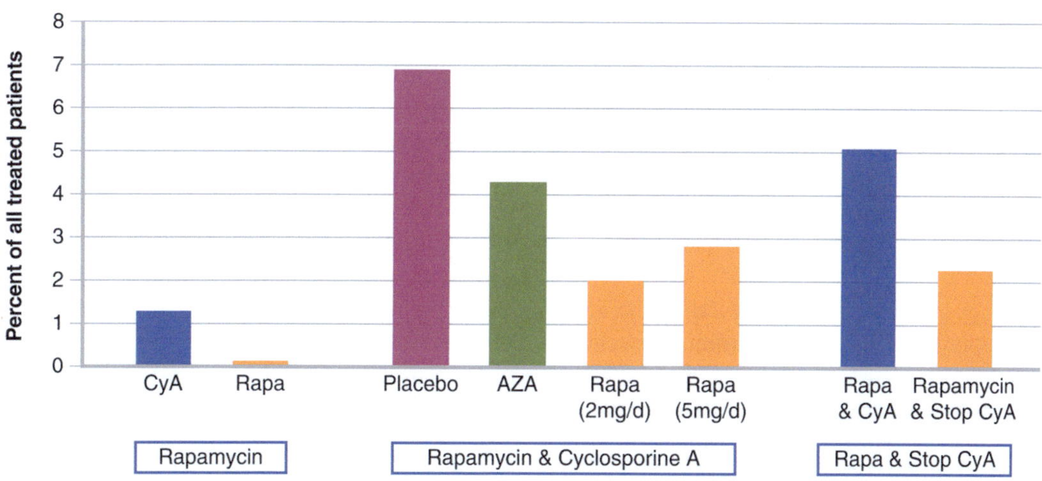

Fig. 4.2 Skin cancer incidence in registration studies for rapamycin. Skin cancer was not a primary objective in these studies but assessed as a secondary parameter

Some registration studies for sirolimus reported as secondary outcome parameters a lower skin cancer incidence in OTR on sirolimus compared to those on calcineurin inhibitors (with either first-time therapy [50] or after switching [51–53]).

De Fijter [55] examined the use of the mTOR inhibitors in 53 renal transplant recipients developing skin cancer post transplantation. In 37 patients, epithelial skin cancer regressed. The tolerability of both sirolimus and everolimus seems to be good with minimal adverse events, pointing to mTOR inhibitors as a tool in the management of epithelial skin cancer in OTR [47, 48, 54, 55]. Existing SCCs post transplantation demonstrated a reduction of thickness and vascularization after the switch from CNI to sirolimus [56].

The CONVERT trial examined 555 renal allograft recipients who converted to a CNI-free and sirolimus-based therapy. Two years after the switch from CNI to sirolimus, the conversion group suffered fewer malignancies in general, including NMSC, compared to those who continued on CNIs (2.2 % vs. 7.7 %; $p<0.001$). The graft and patient survival were equal in both groups [52].

A 2012 published study with 86 kidney transplant recipients was about in line with the CONVERT trial. The NMSC rate was reduced with sirolimus (1.31 vs. 2.48 lesions/patient-year; $p=0.022$). Squamous cell carcinoma occurred at a lower rate in the sirolimus versus CNI group ($p=0.038$), while the rate of basal cell carcinoma was indifferent. A lower percentage of OTR on sirolimus showed new or recurrent NMSC (56.4 % vs. 80.9 %; $p=0.015$) or new squamous cell carcinoma (41.0 % vs. 70.2 %; $p=0.006$) [51].

The TUMORAPA study observed kidney transplant recipients on CNI therapy with at least one cutaneous squamous cell carcinoma. One group was converted to sirolimus, while the other continued CNI treatment. Converting the immunosuppression from CNI to sirolimus resulted in a reduced risk for subsequent skin cancers, with disease-free survival longer for OTR on sirolimus than on CNI. In summary, 14 patients (22 %) on sirolimus developed new squamous cell carcinomas (6 after stopping sirolimus), while 22 (39 %) of OTR on CNI did so (median time until onset, 15 vs. 7 months; $P=0.02$). The relative risk for SCC in OTR on sirolimus stood at 0.56 (95 % confidence interval, 0.32–0.98). Kidney graft function did not change in the either study group. Switching from CNI to sirolimus showed therefore an antitumoral effect among transplant recipients with previous squamous cell carcinoma [53].

The data suggest that the earlier the conversion occurs after an initial diagnosis of cutaneous squamous cell carcinoma, the greater the efficacy. The effect was clear for those OTR with a first SCC (hazard ratio, 0.03; 95 % CI, 0.0–0.91) but not for those with more than one SCC (hazard ratio, 0.67; 95 % CI, 0.29–1.54) [53].

A small German study investigated if mTOR inhibitors could also be a safe immunosuppressive strategy for renal transplant recipients without having had a previous skin cancer. The study included all forms of histologically confirmed nonmelanoma skin cancer and premalignancies. One year after conversion, NMSC was reported in one out of 16 patients in the sirolimus conversion group compared with eight out of 17 in the control group ($p=0.0176$). The one malignancy in the sirolimus group was a BCC. The control-group patients were kept on their preexisting medication (9xAza, 6xMMF, 1x tacrolimus, 1x cyclosporine; all in combination with prednisone). In the control arm, five SCCs, two Bowen carcinomas, and one BCC were histologically confirmed [57].

The RESCUE (Recurrent Cutaneous Squamous Cell Carcinoma Under Rapamune) study tried to find out whether switching to sirolimus-based immunosuppression in renal transplant recipients could confirm a risk reduction of new invasive SCCs. Surprisingly, the RESCUE study failed to attest an improvement in risk reduction for NMSC. The study disclosed that switching to sirolimus did not bring a benefit for SCC-free survival time after 2 years. One hundred and fifty-five renal transplant recipients with at least one histologically proven SCC were randomly divided into two groups: patients converting to sirolimus versus patients continuing original immunosuppression. In the first year after the switch to sirolimus, an effect on SCC was seen in these RTR with one SCC only. On multivariable analysis, OTR on sirolimus had a hazard ratio of 0.76 (95 % CI, 0.48–1.2; $P = 0.255$) for a second SCC over the 2-year follow-up with an insignificant 24 % risk reduction for at least one subsequent invasive SCC. In conclusion, the study displays a benefit in switching early to sirolimus-based maintenance therapy, but the switch from CNI to sirolimus should be done as early as possible in OTRs with cutaneous carcinomas to prevent further SCC in the future for these patients [58].

Switching from CNI to sirolimus for its antitumoral benefits may be considered for kidney transplant recipients without proteinuria no less than 6 months post-transplant after the surgical wounds have completely healed [3].

Myelosuppression and hyperlipidemia are the most reported adverse effects of sirolimus. Because of multiple other adverse effects like impaired wound healing, pneumonitis, thrombotic microangiopathy, edema, aphthous ulceration, and decreased testosterone levels in male patients and because graft survival on sirolimus as primary immunosuppression following kidney transplantation was inferior to CNI in the first year post-transplant, sirolimus is unlikely to be used as monotherapy shortly after transplantation [59].

Proteinuria – another side effect – could be seen in renal transplant recipients and has to be considered before converting from CNI to a sirolimus-based regime. Three hundred and sixty days after the conversion, mean proteinuria increased significantly from 0.37–0.34 to 1.81–1.73 g/34 h ($p < 0.005$) in contrast to the control group where no increase was detected. This proteinuria was reversible and interestingly only visible in patients with preexisting proteinuria before the conversion [60].

The TUMORAPA study has displayed that mTOR inhibitors have a stronger effect on cutaneous squamous cell carcinomas than basal cell carcinomas. Two years after conversion to sirolimus, the SCC:BCC ratio in renal transplant recipients was reduced from 3.9:1 to 1.4:1 [53]. This stronger antitumoral effect of mTOR inhibitors in SCC could be due to the higher cytoplasmic expression of phosphorylated-mTOR in SCC than in BCC. Clinical observation suggests that more frequent expressions of p-mTOR are in line with a higher antitumoral effect of mTOR inhibitors. Data on p-mTOR expression in NMSC are limited [61].

Cells outside the immune system and colon cancer cell lines showed relative resistance to sirolimus, where only very high drug levels of 100–400 mg/kg/d intraperitoneally impaired proliferation. Therefore, the inhibitory effect of normal immunosuppressive doses of sirolimus on tumor growth is probably not due to an antiproliferative effect on tumor cells. Guba et al. confirmed that sirolimus-treated mouse models displayed a decrease of tumor angiogenesis and subsequent tumor growth [29].

4.5 Summary

There are multiple ways to reduce NMSC in OTRs, not only based on minimizing immunosuppression. Currently, mTOR inhibitors are of great interest. It is challenging to find the accurate moment to convert to an mTOR inhibitor to maintain graft function without inducing NMSC in OTRs. The profits and disadvantages of switching to an mTOR inhibitor must be evaluated for every single patient individually. In our opinion, switching to rapamycin should be advised for transplant patients with squamous cell carcinoma early, owing to the high risk of subsequent skin lesions.

There are three important factors in the pathogenesis of posttransplant skin SCCs:

- Preexisting solar damage accumulating UV-dependent mutations in, for example, TP53 and HRAS is like an avalanche waiting to be triggered by reduced tumor surveillance of the immune system following transplantation.
- Selective and direct effects of immunosuppressants on keratinocytes contributing to skin cancer formation such as an inhibition of p53 by ATF3 upregulation.
- Bystander effects where immunosuppression allows infectious agents such as HPV to increase carcinogenesis by impaired DNA repair in keratinocytes and inhibition of Notch

Table 4.2 Possible actions to reduce SCC formation in OTRs

Daily photoprotection
Discontinuation of photosensitizing drugs
Early treatment of field cancerization and actinic keratosis
Treatment of human papillomavirus at an early stage
Treat chronic inflammation which contributes to SCC formation
Reduce immunosuppression (lowest possible dose)
Reduction from triple to single immunosuppressive therapy
Switch immunosuppressive drugs CNI to mTOR inhibitors
Switch immunosuppressive drugs AZA to MMF

following UV damage which is discussed in the respective chapter in more detail.

The interventions resulting from these steps in cutaneous carcinogenesis are as follows:

- Constant sun protection to prevent the accumulation of further actinic damage in OTR, where preexisting long-term genetic field defects are largely irreversible.
- Switching from CNI to mTOR and from AZA to MMF in particular early in cutaneous carcinogenesis. These dermatologically helpful changes must be balanced in respect to graft function and other adverse effects.
- Targeting DNA repair and Notch by HPV vaccination and development of novel agents. While these agents are currently not available for clinical use, evolving field cancerization can be addressed by recurring treatment cycles with imiquimod, 5-fluorouracil, ingenol mebutate, photodynamic therapy, and systemic acitretin (Table 4.2).

References

1. Kempf W, Mertz KD, Hofbauer GF, Tinguely M. Skin cancer in organ transplant recipients. Pathobiology. 2013;80(6):302–9.
2. Hofbauer GF, Bouwes Bavinck JN, Euvrard S. Organ transplantation and skin cancer: basic problems and new perspectives. Exp Dermatol. 2010;19(6):473–82.
3. Zwald FO, Brown M. Skin cancer in solid organ transplant recipients: advances in therapy and management: part I. Epidemiology of skin cancer in solid organ transplant recipients. J Am Acad Dermatol. 2011;65(2):253–61; quiz 262.
4. Euvrard S, Kanitakis J, Pouteil-Noble C, Claudy A, Touraine JL. Skin cancers in organ transplant recipients. Ann Transplant. 1997;2(4):28–32.
5. Connolly K, Manders P, Earls P, Epstein RJ. Papillomavirus-associated squamous skin cancers following transplant immunosuppression: one Notch closer to control. Cancer Treat Rev. 2014;40(2):205–14.
6. Ulrich C, Schmook T, Sachse MM, Sterry W, Stockfleth E. Comparative epidemiology and pathogenic factors for nonmelanoma skin cancer in organ transplant patients. Dermatol Surg. 2004;30(4 Pt 2):622–7.
7. Mehrany K, Weenig RH, Lee KK, Pittelkow MR, Otley CC. Increased metastasis and mortality from cutaneous squamous cell carcinoma in patients with chronic lymphocytic leukemia. J Am Acad Dermatol. 2005;53(6):1067–71.
8. Euvrard S, Kanitakis J, Claudy A. Skin cancers after organ transplantation. N Engl J Med. 2003;348(17):1681–91.
9. Webb MC, Compton F, Andrews PA, Koffman CG. Skin tumours posttransplantation: a retrospective analysis of 28 years' experience at a single centre. Transplant Proc. 1997;29(1–2):828–30.
10. Muehleisen B, Pazhenkottil A, French LE, Hofbauer GF. Nonmelanoma skin cancer in organ transplant recipients: increase without delay after transplant and subsequent acceleration. JAMA Dermatol. 2013;149(5):618–20.
11. Caforio AL, Fortina AB, Piaserico S, et al. Skin cancer in heart transplant recipients: risk factor analysis and relevance of immunosuppressive therapy. Circulation. 2000;102(19 Suppl 3):III222–7.
12. Euvrard S, Kanitakis J. Skin cancers after liver transplantation: what to do? J Hepatol. 2006;44(1):27–32.
13. Jensen P, Hansen S, Møller B, et al. Skin cancer in kidney and heart transplant recipients and different long-term immunosuppressive therapy regimens. J Am Acad Dermatol. 1999;40(2 Pt 1):177–86.
14. Euvrard S, Kanitakis J, Pouteil-Noble C, et al. Comparative epidemiologic study of premalignant and malignant epithelial cutaneous lesions developing after kidney and heart transplantation. J Am Acad Dermatol. 1995;33(2 Pt 1):222–9.
15. Ducloux D, Carron PL, Rebibou JM, et al. CD4 lymphocytopenia as a risk factor for skin cancers in renal transplant recipients. Transplantation. 1998;65(9):1270–2.
16. Abou Ayache R, Thierry A, Bridoux F, et al. Long-term maintenance of calcineurin inhibitor monotherapy reduces the risk for squamous cell carcinomas after kidney transplantation compared with bi- or tritherapy. Transplant Proc. 2007;39(8):2592–4.
17. Glover MT, Deeks JJ, Raftery MJ, Cunningham J, Leigh IM. Immunosuppression and risk of non-melanoma skin cancer in renal transplant recipients. Lancet. 1997;349(9049):398.
18. Watorek E, Boratynska M, Smolska D, Patrzalek D, Klinger M. Malignancy after renal transplantation in the new era of immunosuppression. Ann Transplant. 2011;16(2):14–8.

19. Reynolds NJ, Al-Daraji WI. Calcineurin inhibitors and sirolimus: mechanisms of action and applications in dermatology. Clin Exp Dermatol. 2002;27:555–61.
20. Karagas MR, Cushing GL, Greenberg ER, Mott LA, Spencer SK, Nierenberg DW. Non-melanoma skin cancers and glucocorticoid therapy. Br J Cancer. 2001;85(5):683–6.
21. Sørensen HT, Mellemkjaer L, Nielsen GL, Baron JA, Olsen JH, Karagas MR. Skin cancers and non-Hodgkin lymphoma among users of systemic glucocorticoids: a population-based cohort study. J Natl Cancer Inst. 2004;96(9):709–11.
22. Jensen A, Thomsen HF, Engebjerg MC, et al. Use of oral glucocorticoids and risk of skin cancer and non-Hodgkin's lymphoma: a population-based case–control study. Br J Cancer. 2009;100(1):200–5.
23. Berg D, Otley CC. Skin cancer in organ transplant recipients: epidemiology, pathogenesis, and management. J Am Acad Dermatol. 2002;47(1):1–17; quiz 18–20.
24. Dantal J, Hourmant M, Cantarovich D, et al. Effect of long-term immunosuppression in kidney-graft recipients on cancer incidence: randomised comparison of two cyclosporin regimens. Lancet. 1998;351(9103):623–8.
25. Bichari W, Bartiromo M, Mohey H, et al. Significant risk factors for occurrence of cancer after renal transplantation: a single center cohort study of 1265 cases. Transplant Proc. 2009;41(2):672–3.
26. Hojo M, Morimoto T, Maluccio M, et al. Cyclosporine induces cancer progression by a cell-autonomous mechanism. Nature. 1999;397(6719):530–4.
27. Maluccio M, Sharma V, Lagman M, et al. Tacrolimus enhances transforming growth factor-beta1 expression and promotes tumor progression. Transplantation. 2003;76(3):597–602.
28. Mohamed MA, Robertson H, Booth TA, Balupuri S, Kirby JA, Talbot D. TGF-beta expression in renal transplant biopsies: a comparative study between cyclosporin-A and tacrolimus. Transplantation. 2000;69(5):1002–5.
29. Guba M, von Breitenbuch P, Steinbauer M, et al. Rapamycin inhibits primary and metastatic tumor growth by antiangiogenesis: involvement of vascular endothelial growth factor. Nat Med. 2002;8(2):128–35.
30. Norman KG, Canter JA, Shi M, Milne GL, Morrow JD, Sligh JE. Cyclosporine A suppresses keratinocyte cell death through MPTP inhibition in a model for skin cancer in organ transplant recipients. Mitochondrion. 2010;10(2):94–101.
31. Yarosh DB, Pena AV, Nay SL, Canning MT, Brown DA. Calcineurin inhibitors decrease DNA repair and apoptosis in human keratinocytes following ultraviolet B irradiation. J Invest Dermatol. 2005;125(5):1020–5.
32. Wu X, Nguyen BC, Dziunycz P, et al. Opposing roles for calcineurin and ATF3 in squamous skin cancer. Nature. 2010;465(7296):368–72.
33. Lindelöf B, Dal H, Wolk K, Malmborg N. Cutaneous squamous cell carcinoma in organ transplant recipients: a study of the Swedish cohort with regard to tumor site. Arch Dermatol. 2005;141(4):447–51.
34. Dziunycz PJ, Lefort K, Wu X, et al. The oncogene ATF3 is potentiated by cyclosporine A and ultraviolet light A. J Invest Dermatol. 2014;134(7):1998–2004.
35. Ingvar A, Smedby KE, Lindelöf B, et al. Immunosuppressive treatment after solid organ transplantation and risk of post-transplant cutaneous squamous cell carcinoma. Nephrol Dial Transplant. 2010;25(8):2764–71.
36. van den Reek JM, van Lümig PP, Janssen M, et al. Increased incidence of squamous cell carcinoma of the skin after long-term treatment with azathioprine in patients with auto-immune inflammatory rheumatic diseases. J Eur Acad Dermatol Venereol. 2014;28(1):27–33.
37. O'Donovan P, Perrett CM, Zhang X, et al. Azathioprine and UVA light generate mutagenic oxidative DNA damage. Science. 2005;309(5742):1871–4.
38. de Graaf YG, Rebel H, Elghalbzouri A, et al. More epidermal p53 patches adjacent to skin carcinomas in renal transplant recipients than in immunocompetent patients: the role of azathioprine. Exp Dermatol. 2008;17(4):349–55.
39. Kelly GE, Meikle W, Sheil AG. Effects of immunosuppressive therapy on the induction of skin tumors by ultraviolet irradiation in hairless mice. Transplantation. 1987;44(3):429–34.
40. Hofbauer GF, Attard NR, Harwood CA, et al. Reversal of UVA skin photosensitivity and DNA damage in kidney transplant recipients by replacing azathioprine. Am J Transplant. 2012;12(1):218–25.
41. Keogh A. Long-term benefits of mycophenolate mofetil after heart transplantation. Transplantation. 2005;79(3 Suppl):S45–6.
42. O'Neill JO, Edwards LB, Taylor DO. Mycophenolate mofetil and risk of developing malignancy after orthotopic heart transplantation: analysis of the transplant registry of the International Society for Heart and Lung Transplantation. J Heart Lung Transplant. 2006;25(10):1186–91.
43. Robson R, Cecka JM, Opelz G, Budde M, Sacks S. Prospective registry-based observational cohort study of the long-term risk of malignancies in renal transplant patients treated with mycophenolate mofetil. Am J Transplant. 2005;5(12):2954–60.
44. Krötz F, Keller M, Derflinger S, et al. Mycophenolate acid inhibits endothelial NAD(P)H oxidase activity and superoxide formation by a Rac1-dependent mechanism. Hypertension. 2007;49(1):201–8.
45. Geissler EK, Schlitt HJ, Thomas G. mTOR, cancer and transplantation. Am J Transplant. 2008;8(11):2212–8.
46. Euvrard S, Ulrich C, Lefrancois N. Immunosuppressants and skin cancer in transplant patients: focus on rapamycin. Dermatol Surg. 2004;30(4 Pt 2):628–33.
47. Kauffman HM, Cherikh WS, Cheng Y, Hanto DW, Kahan BD. Maintenance immunosuppression with target-of-rapamycin inhibitors is associated with a reduced incidence of de novo malignancies. Transplantation. 2005;80(7):883–9.

48. Yakupoglu YK, Buell JF, Woodle S, Kahan BD. Individualization of immunosuppressive therapy. III. Sirolimus associated with a reduced incidence of malignancy. Transplant Proc. 2006;38(2):358–61.
49. Carroll RP, Hester J, Wood KJ, Harden PN. Conversion to sirolimus in kidney transplant recipients with squamous cell cancer and changes in immune phenotype. Nephrol Dial Transplant. 2013;28(2):462–5.
50. Mathew T, Kreis H, Friend P. Two-year incidence of malignancy in sirolimus-treated renal transplant recipients: results from five multicenter studies. Clin Transplant. 2004;18(4):446–9.
51. Campbell SB, Walker R, Tai SS, Jiang Q, Russ GR. Randomized controlled trial of sirolimus for renal transplant recipients at high risk for nonmelanoma skin cancer. Am J Transplant. 2012;12(5):1146–56.
52. Alberú J, Pascoe MD, Campistol JM, et al. Lower malignancy rates in renal allograft recipients converted to sirolimus-based, calcineurin inhibitor-free immunotherapy: 24-month results from the CONVERT trial. Transplantation. 2011;92(3):303–10.
53. Euvrard S, Morelon E, Rostaing L, et al. Sirolimus and secondary skin-cancer prevention in kidney transplantation. N Engl J Med. 2012;367(4):329–39.
54. Fernández A, Marcén R, Pascual J, et al. Conversion from calcineurin inhibitors to everolimus in kidney transplant recipients with malignant neoplasia. Transplant Proc. 2006;38(8):2453–5.
55. de Fijter JW. Use of proliferation signal inhibitors in non-melanoma skin cancer following renal transplantation. Nephrol Dial Transplant. 2007;22 Suppl 1:i23–6.
56. Rival-Tringali AL, Euvrard S, Decullier E, Claudy A, Faure M, Kanitakis J. Conversion from calcineurin inhibitors to sirolimus reduces vascularization and thickness of post-transplant cutaneous squamous cell carcinomas. Anticancer Res. 2009;29(6):1927–32.
57. Salgo R, Gossmann J, Schöfer H, et al. Switch to a sirolimus-based immunosuppression in long-term renal transplant recipients: reduced rate of (pre-) malignancies and nonmelanoma skin cancer in a prospective, randomized, assessor-blinded, controlled clinical trial. Am J Transplant. 2010;10(6): 1385–93.
58. Hoogendijk-van den Akker JM, Harden PN, Hoitsma AJ, et al. Two-year randomized controlled prospective trial converting treatment of stable renal transplant recipients with cutaneous invasive squamous cell carcinomas to sirolimus. J Clin Oncol. 2013;31(10):1317–23.
59. Augustine JJ, Bodziak KA, Hricik DE. Use of sirolimus in solid organ transplantation. Drugs. 2007;67(3): 369–91.
60. van den Akker JM, Wetzels JF, Hoitsma AJ. Proteinuria following conversion from azathioprine to sirolimus in renal transplant recipients. Kidney Int. 2006;70(7):1355–7.
61. Karayannopoulou G, Euvrard S, Kanitakis J. Differential expression of p-mTOR in cutaneous basal and squamous cell carcinomas likely explains their different response to mTOR inhibitors in organ-transplant recipients. Anticancer Res. 2013;33(9):3711–4.
62. Euvrard S, Kanitakis J, Decullier E, et al. Subsequent skin cancers in kidney and heart transplant recipients after the first squamous cell carcinoma. Transplantation. 2006;81(8):1093–100.

Advances in Photodynamic Therapy for the Treatment of Malignant and Premalignant Lesions in Transplant Dermatology

5

Jason Michael Rizzo and Nathalie C. Zeitouni

Contents

J.M. Rizzo, BS, PhD
Department of Biochemistry, SUNY Buffalo School of Medicine & Biomedical Sciences, Buffalo, NY, USA
e-mail: jrizzo6@buffalo.edu

N.C. Zeitouni, MDCM, FRCPC (✉)
Department of Dermatology, Roswell Park Cancer Institute, Buffalo, NY, USA
e-mail: Nathalie.Zeitouni@RoswellPark.org

5.1 Background

Photodynamic therapy (PDT) is a field-based therapy with well-documented clinical efficacy in the treatment of nonmelanoma skin cancer (NMSC) and its precursor lesions, i.e., actinic keratosis (AK) and Bowen's disease (BD) [1–3]. There are three major components of PDT: a photosensitizer (PS), a light source, and oxygen. Individually each component is not toxic, but combined they initiate a photochemical reaction which generates singlet oxygen. In turn, this reactive oxygen species can rapidly cause significant toxicity leading to cell death [4].

The antitumor effects on PDT consist of both direct and indirect mechanisms. Direct cell death occurs through apoptosis and necrosis secondary to induced phototoxicity. Indirect damage occurs as a result of phototoxic damage to the tumor vasculature and development of an inflammatory response, predominantly of an innate immune nature [4, 5]. Overall, the relative contribution of each of these inter-related mechanisms is highly variable and depends on factors including the type, dose, and timing of PS and light sources employed [6, 7]. The choice of optimal combinations of these treatment parameters is crucial for successful PDT and remains an active area of interdisciplinary research [8].

There are two types of PSs employed in PDT, systemic and topical, and several hundred compounds are currently under investigation [6]. In oncology, PSs are typically based on a tetrapyrrole

F. Zwald, M.D. Brown (eds.), *Advances in Transplant Dermatology: Clinical and Practical Implications*,
DOI 10.1007/978-3-319-12445-2_5,

structure analogous to the protoporphyrin contained in hemoglobin. In dermatology, PDT is primarily delivered through the use of the topical PS 5-aminolevulinic acid (ALA) or its methylated ester, methyl aminolevulinate (MAL). Only ALA is currently available in the USA and FDA approved, while MAL is widely used in Europe and Canada. Both ALA and MAL are precursors in heme biosynthesis and act as prodrugs in the skin, converted into photoactivatable porphyrins, including protoporphyrin IX (PpIX) [2]. The excitability of these molecules coupled with their tumor-localizing properties underscores their utility as PS agents [9]. Importantly, none of the clinically approved PDs accumulate in cell nuclei, limiting their carcinogenic potential [4].

In terms of light sources, there are two types: lasers and non-laser, both of which have shown similar clinical efficacy [10]. Lasers used in PDT include an argon-pumped dye, diode, pulse dye laser, Nd:Yag pumped dye, as well as the gold vapor laser. The advantage of lasers is the ability to modify the energy. Non-laser light sources include light-emitting diode (LED) arrays and blue light fluorescent tubes which are widely commercially available for PDT. Other non-laser light sources include intense pulse light and filtered halogen/xenon arc lamps. Depth of tissue penetration is related to wavelength, and red light may be more suitable for deeper lesions, since it has a longer wavelength than blue light. Only LED and blue light are currently FDA approved for use with PDT.

5.2 PDT in OTRs

5.2.1 Overview

Clinical applications for the use of PDT that have shown successful outcomes include actinic keratosis (AK), Bowen's disease (BD), and basal cell carcinoma (BCC). Many other conditions have been treated with PDT with mixed results including extramammary Paget's disease, cutaneous T-cell lymphoma, squamous cell carcinoma (SCC), and Kaposi's sarcoma. Here we review the evidence for use of PDT in the organ transplant recipient (OTR) population.

OTRs are at significant risk for the development of NMSC. They have between a 65- and 200-fold increased risk for the development of SCC and a 10-fold increased risk of developing BCC compared to the general population [11–14]. These patients are also at increased risk for the development of precancerous lesions including AK and BD, with AKs demonstrating a greater propensity toward malignant transformation into invasive SCC [13, 15]. Overall, NMSC and its precursor lesions tend to be more numerous, diffusely located, recurrent, and aggressive in OTRs compared to immunocompetent patients (Fig. 5.1) [16–21]. Not surprisingly, cutaneous malignancy is therefore the leading cause of morbidity and mortality in this immunosuppressed patient population. Given this significant disease burden, a great deal of interest has focused on the treatment and prevention of NMSC in OTRs. As a convenient and economical field-based therapy capable of treating large areas or multiple lesions simultaneously with excellent cosmetic outcomes, the use PDT has been explored as both a primary modality for and in prevention of NMSC, and its precursors, in the OTR population.

5.2.2 Primary Treatment of NMSC and Precursors

As a primary treatment modality, studies with PDT and OTR have mainly focused on AK and BD (see Table 5.1). One of the first reports was a prospective trial using ALA in 20 OTRs and 20 controls. The average area of AK/BD was 3×4 cm in diameter, and 1–2 sessions were performed using a noncoherent light source. The authors found a high initial complete response rate (CRR) at 4 weeks of 86 % for OTR vs 94 % for controls using PDT. The long-term clearance at 12 weeks decreased for both groups to 68 % vs 89 % and at 48 weeks was 48 % vs 72 % but was significantly lower in the OTR group [29].

Several other studies have since been reported using MAL as the topical photosensitizer for PDT. Dragieva et al. treated 17 OTRs with multiple AKs with 2 consecutive treatments 1 week apart with a noncoherent light source and found a

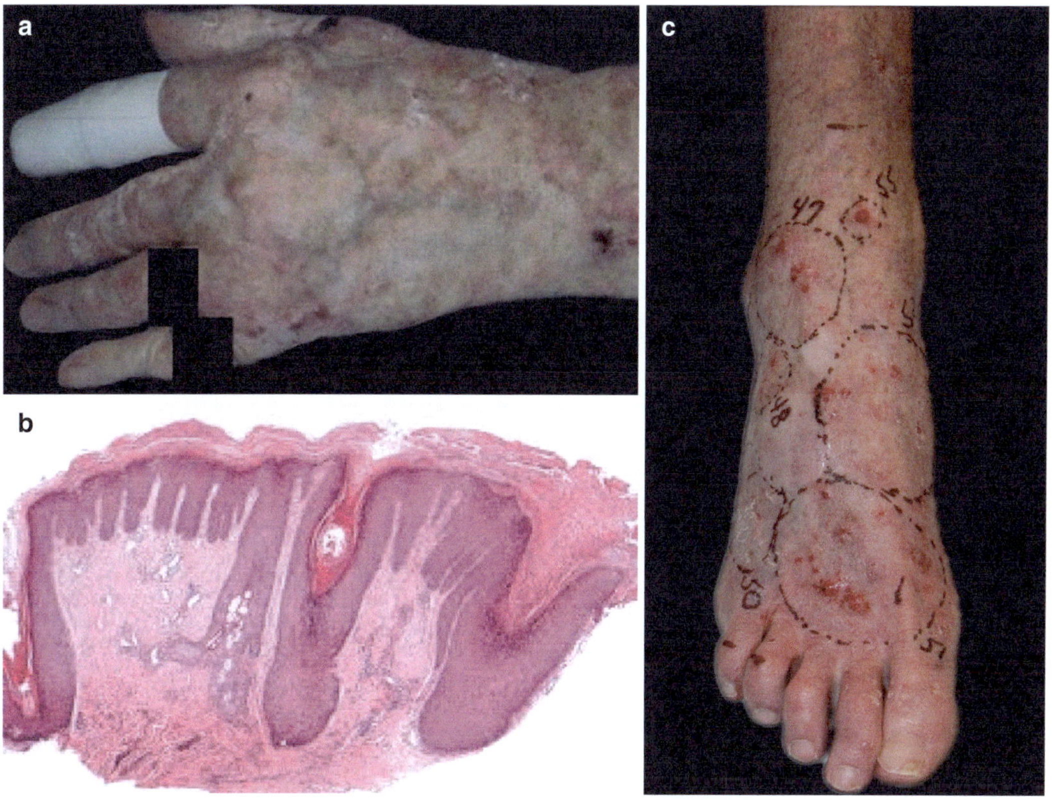

Fig. 5.1 Examples of extensive disease involvement and difficult-to-treat lesions in OTRs. (**a**) Gross morphology of diffuse AKs with hyperkeratosis populating the left dorsal hand of an OTR. Hyperkeratotic lesions inhibit uptake of photosensitizing agents during PDT protocols and may contribute to inferior efficacy if not addressed by appropriate pretreatment considerations (see Table 5.3). (**b**) Photomicrograph of H&E staining illustrating underlying hyperkeratosis for lesions depicted in (a). (**c**) Gross morphology of large widespread lesions on the right dorsal foot seen in an OTR with Bowen's disease

90 % response rate at 3 months [23]. Piaserico et al. also treated 15 OTRs with multiple AKs unresponsive to conventional therapy with 2 sessions 2 weeks apart with a red light and found an overall CR of 71 % at 3 months [24]. These authors also found a lower response rate for the hands 40 % vs the scalp and face 72 %. In their patients, PDT was associated with severe pain in 47 %. In a prospective study in 16 OTRs with AK and photodamage, Hasson and colleagues found a CR of 100 % at 12 and 24 weeks, using 1–2 sessions of red light. They also saw 62.5 % improved photodamage in those patients [26].

Compared to AK and BD, there are more limited case reports and short series regarding PDT use in treatment of superficial and small nodular BCCs (sBCC and nBCC, respectively) in OTRs (see Table 5.1). Schleier and colleagues were the first to explore the use of PDT for primary treatment of BCC, treating 21 clinically diagnosed facial BCCs in 5 OTRs, multifocally, with topical application of ALA using thermogel followed by a single treatment of PDT with a diode laser [22]. The authors reported an excellent response to therapy for all tumors, with 20/21 showing a CRR at 12 weeks and subsequent success from repeated treatment of the sole nonresponding tumor. Two other reports have since followed, examining the role of MAL-PDT in the treatment of sBCC and nBCC. Mean follow-up varied between 12 and 22.6 months. Only 1/18 recurrence was noted, and it appears that PDT may be effective in the short term in these patients [31, 32].

Table 5.1 Summary of studies of PDT in OTR for primary treatment of NMSC and precursor lesions

Lesion type	OTR (*n*)	OTR type	# lesions (areas)	PS (dose %)	PS time (h)	Light source	Light dose (J/cm^2)	Intensity (mW/cm^2)	Study design	CRR	Follow-up (weeks)	Reference
AK	3	Heart, kidney	8	ALA (40)	3–5	635 nm diode laser ×1	120	100	Prospective case series	88 %	12	[22]
AK	17	Heart, kidney	129 (17)	MAL (NOS)[b]	3	Incoherent visible light 630–730 nm ×2	75	80	Randomized, placebo-controlled trial	76 % lesional areas	16	[23]
AK	15	Kidney	245 (33)	MAL (NOS)[b]	3	633 nm red light ×2	37	NOS	Prospective case series	64 % lesional areas	12	[24]
AK	81	Heart, kidney, lung, liver	385	MAL (16)[b]	3	630 nm red light ×1–5	37	NOS	Randomized, intrapatient controlled comparative trial (vs cryotherapy)	77 %	12	[25]
AK	16	Heart, kidney, liver	NOS[a]	MAL (16)[b]	3	635 nm red light ×1–2	37	NOS	Prospective case series	100 %	12 and 24	[26]
AK	12	NOS	59	MAL (16)[c]	3	NOS ×3	90	NOS	Prospective case series	100 % and 83 %	16 and 36	[27]
AK	10	Heart, kidney, liver	335	MAL (16)[d]	3	632 nm red light ×1	37	NOS	Randomized half-side comparative trial	73 %	16	[28]
AK and BD	20	Heart, kidney	44	ALA (20)[e]	5	Incoherent visible light NOS ×1	75	80	Prospective case series	68 %	12	[29]
AK and BD	8	Kidney, liver	NOS (9)	MAL (16)[b]	3	633 nm red light ×2	75	80	Randomized, intrapatient controlled comparative trial (vs 5-FU)	89 %	12 and 24	[30]

KA	1	Heart	11	ALA (40)	3–5	635 nm diode laser ×1	120	100	Prospective case series	100 %	12	[22]
SCC	2	Kidney	2	ALA (40)	3–5	635 nm diode laser ×1	120	100	Prospective case series	0 %	12	[22]
Mostly sBCC	5	Heart, kidney, BMT	21	ALA (40)	3–5	635 nm diode laser ×1	120	100	Prospective case series	95 %	12	[22]
Small nBCC	1	Liver	1	MAL (16)[b]	3	633 nm red light ×2	75	80	Case report	100 %	12	[31]
sBCC and nBCC	18	Heart, kidney, lung, liver, pancreas	18	MAL (NOS)[f]	3	630 nm red light ×2	37	NOS	Prospective case series	94 %	26.2[g]	[32]

AFLX ablative fractional CO_2 laser, *CRR* complete response rate, *NOS* not otherwise specified, *PS* photosensitizer

[a]Face and scalp only

[b]Pretreatment curettage

[c]Pretreatment microneedling

[d]Pretreatment AFLX

[e]Pretreatment curettage or salicylic acid

[f]Pretreatment NOS

[g]Average follow-up

5.2.3 Pretreatment Considerations

In immunocompetent patients, PDT has been shown to be as effective and often superior to the use of conventional treatments for AK and BD, such as cryotherapy and topical 5-fluorouracil (5-FU) cream [4]. PDT, however, offers additional advantages in that it tends to produce improved cosmesis and can be better tolerated. For example, in one study, comparing MAL-PDT to cryotherapy, both investigator and patient assessment were higher for PDT in terms of overall cosmetic outcome [33]. Similar findings have been documented in limited head-to-head comparisons in the OTR population. In a randomized intrapatient comparative study between MAL-PDT and 5-FU cream, 8 OTRs with AK/BD were treated with 1–2 sessions of PDT 1 week apart for 5 weeks or 5-FU BID for 3 weeks. Overall, PDT proved to be significantly more effective in the treatment of epidermal dysplasia with a CRR of 89 % compared to 11 % for 5-FU. Additionally, cosmetic outcome and patient preference were again superior with PDT, but the pain intensity was also higher with PDT [30].

Despite similar efficacy to conventional therapies within a given patient population, PDT has demonstrated overall lower response rates to the treatment of AK/BD when comparing OTRs to non-immunocompromised [14]. Interestingly, the discordance of PDT response between immunosuppressed and immunocompetent patients has not been seen in limited studies of BCC. A recent retrospective case series review of 322 BCCs in 103 patients by Collier and Lear found no significant difference in BCC recurrence following PDT in OTR versus non-transplant patients, regardless of lesional site location [34]. Similarly, the largest prospective study to date of sBCC and nBCC, by Guleng and Helsing, also showed PDT to be equally effective in OTR and immunocompetent patients [32]. Among the many factors contributing to the inferior efficacy of PDT in the OTR population for AK/BD, variance in photosensitization is a major culprit. Photosensitization is related to both optimal uptake of the photosensitizing drug and adequate light penetration. In OTR, uptake is frequently limited by the increased hyperkeratosis as evidenced by the thick AK/BD seen in the patients (Fig. 5.1a, b) [14]. Attempts to address this limitation have aimed to increase photosensitizer penetration including the use of one or combined methods prior to therapy: curettage, debulking, keratolytics, microdermabrasion, laser ablation, 5-FU cream, fractional CO_2 laser, and microneedling.

Combined MAL-PDT and pretreatment of tumor cells with 5-FU cream have been used in both in vitro and murine in vivo studies. Pretreatment with 5-FU has been shown to increase 3–4 times photosensitizer drug accumulation compared to non-pretreated cells. In 12 OTRs with a total of 48 AK/BD on the face and scalp, Maytin and colleagues had one group of patients use 5-FU cream as pretreatment for 6 days and then undergo MAL-PDT with a red light source and compared these patients to patients who only had PDT. In the pretreatment group Pp IX levels were measured and found to be higher than in the PDT group alone. At 3–12-month follow-up, patients in the pretreatment group also had reduced new lesion formation [35].

PDT has also been combined with the fractional CO_2 laser in an attempt to increase effectiveness. In one report, immunocompetent patients underwent ablative fractional CO_2 resurfacing for AKs and then were applied with MAL for 3 h and treated with a red light. Combined treatment at 3 months was more effective with a CR of 88–100 % vs the PDT alone with a CR of 59–80 %. Improved photodamage was also seen in the combined group, but there were also more side effects including pain and pigmentation changes [36].

PDT combined with the ablative fractional laser (AFXL) has been used in a group of 10 OTRs with a total of 680 AKs and 409 wartlike lesions (WLL) on the hands, difficult-to-treat areas. All patients underwent 2 passes of AFXL on both hands. One group of patients then underwent MAL-PDT, while the other group had no further treatment. For AKs, the group with AFXL plus PDT had a CR of 73 % vs 31 % in the AFXL-alone group. For WLL the combined group also had a higher CR of 37 % vs 14 % in the AFXL-alone group. The majority of patients required local anesthesia. The authors concluded that AFXL-PDT was effective in OTR, and similar response rates could be achieved in these patients with the combined method as in non-transplant patients [28].

Microneedling prior to PDT has also been attempted in patients in order to achieve higher response rates. In 2 reports in non-immunocompromised patients, patients with photodamage showed improvement with the additional use of microneedling. In patients with AKs, no difference was observed in a small case series using the combined method [37, 38]. Bencini and colleagues had 12 OTRs with 59 AKs undergo microneedling and then MAL-PDT with red light, 3 sessions 2 weeks apart [27]. They found a CR of 83 % at 9 months. Patients tolerated the procedures well, and pain was reduced in further treatment sessions.

5.2.4 Prevention of NMSC and Precursors

The multiplicity and widespread involvement of NMSC and precursor lesions seen in OTRs have spawned a great deal of interest in exploring the effectiveness of PDT for prevention of premalignant and malignant lesions in OTRs (see Table 5.2). Preclinical studies have substantiated this interest, with PDT demonstrating a significant preventative effect in UV-related photocarcinogenesis when delivered to accepted murine models for both SCC and BCC development [42–45].

Wulf and colleagues were the first to present evidence for the concept of PDT use for cancer prevention in immunosuppressed OTRs. In this intrapatient randomized study, a single session of MAL-PDT was delivered to 27 renal transplant patients with AKs and other skin lesions and subsequently compared to an untreated contralateral control area of similar size. Overall, the average time to occurrence for new lesions was significantly longer in the treated areas with a larger percentage of these areas remaining lesion-free after 12 months compared to untreated [39]. A similar, proof-of-concept, study examining the use of PDT in cancer prevention was also conducted in immunocompetent patients by Apalla and colleagues. Utilizing a split-face, placebo-controlled study evaluating a PDT field treatment of facial AKs, they were also able to show a significant delay in the appearance of new AK lesions in PDT-treated regions after 6 months [46, 47].

Continued use of PDT for prevention of NMSC and precursors in OTR has been documented with mixed success in small case series and randomized trials with varied protocols (see Table 5.2). De Graaf and colleagues were the first to examine the effect of PDT on the development of new SCCs with a large randomized intrapatient controlled trial. In this study, 1–2 sessions of blue light ALA-PDT were given to a randomly selected forearm and hand of 40 OTRs, and SCC occurrence was subsequently compared to the contralateral untreated forearm and hand [40]. After 1 year of follow-up, there was a trend in favor of PDT reducing the occurrence of SCC; however, no significant difference was observed at 2 years. No debulking of lesions was performed prior to PDT. In a similarly structured study, Wennberg et al. delivered two sessions of MAL-PDT with red light over 2 weeks at study inception with single treatment follow-ups at 3, 9, and 15 months to 81 OTRs [25]. At 3 months, MAL-PDT was shown to significantly reduce the occurrence of new skin lesions, primarily AKs; however, the significance of this effect was again lost at 27 months follow-up.

Most recently, Willey and colleagues treated 12 OTRs with cyclic ALA-PDT every 4–8 weeks for 2 years [41]. They found a 79 % decrease in new SCC/BD at 12 months and a 95 % decrease compared to baseline at 24 months. Of note, baseline occurrence in this study was defined as the number of SCCs developed during the previous 12–24 months prior to initiation of cyclic PDT.

5.2.5 Treatment Considerations in OTR

Available clinical data lends support for the use of PDT in both the treatment and prevention of NMSC and precursor lesions. Although successful in highlighting the broad potential uses for this therapy in oncology, however, the variable

Table 5.2 Summary of studies of PDT in OTR for NMSC and precursor lesion prevention

OTR (*n*)	OTR type	PS (dose %)	PS time (h)	Light source	Light dose (J/cm^2)	Intensity (mW/cm^2)	Study design	Outcome	Reference
27	Kidney	MAL (16)[a]	3	570–670 nm red light ×1	75	NOS	Randomized, intrapatient controlled comparative trial (vs nontreatment)	Significant reduction in new lesions at 1 year (27 %); mean of 3 months longer until occurrence of new lesions	[39]
40	NOS	ALA (20)	4	400–450 nm violet light ×1–2	5.5–6	NOS	Randomized, intrapatient controlled comparative trial (vs nontreatment)	Nonsignificant reduction in keratotic skin lesions at 1 year No difference at 2 years	[40]
81	Heart, kidney, lung, liver	MAL (16)[b]	3	630 nm red light ×1–5	37	NOS	Randomized, intrapatient controlled comparative trial (vs cryotherapy)	Significant reduction in all new lesions (37 %) primarily AK (46 % reduction) at 12 weeks	[25]
12	Heart, kidney	Cyclic ALA (20)[b]	1	517 nm blue light q 4–8 weeks ×2 years	NOS	10	Prospective case series	Median reduction of 79 and 95 % from baseline at 1 and 2 years	[41]

NOS not otherwise specified, *PS* photosensitizer
[a]Pretreatment surface debridement
[b]Pretreatment curettage

nature of protocols published in the literature, as well as heterogeneity of patient populations examined, has led to mixed results and confounded interpretations (see Tables 5.1 and 5.2). This is particularly true for the case of SCC prevention, where larger, randomized controlled trials failed to reproduce the significant reduction in lesion occurrence identified in earlier case series studies [25, 40]. Importantly, these studies both demonstrated trends toward SCC prevention at secondary end points with shorter-term follow-up, similar to those employed by Willey et al. Specifically, a prospective randomized trial by Wennberg et al. showed a significant reduction in new lesions, including SCC or BCC, at 3 months after two MAL-PDT sessions using red light, with 62 % of treated areas remaining free from new lesions at 12 months [25]. Similarly, de Graaf et al. demonstrated a near significant trend toward SCC prevention at 12- month follow-up in a similarly structured trial using 1–2 treatments with ALA-PDT and blue light [40]. Such differences may be attributable to the lower skin penetration of blue light compared to red. Moreover, these large trials both lacked the more frequent (i.e., cyclical) treatments and pretreatment interventions aimed at maximizing PS penetration, both of which Willey and colleagues employed when finding a significant preventive effect of PDT on SCC development [41]. It is also worth noting that these studies enrolled significantly different patient populations including the severity, number, type, and distribution of lesions examined and treated as well as transplant-specific demographics (i.e., type of transplant, age at transplant, time since transplant, etc.).

Viewed in totality, the aforementioned results highlight the importance of pretreatment considerations as well as the need for more frequent, cyclical treatment interventions when employing PDT for NMSC prevention. Indeed, these findings are further supported by molecular studies, which mirror the clinical response, showing that PDT can reverse or reduce field cancerization but that one single dose is not sufficient to achieve these results [48, 49]. For example, Bagazgoitia and colleagues have shown that two or more treatments of PDT can delay the appearance of AKs, reduce histological features of actinic damage, and decrease expression of early markers of carcinogenesis such as K1-67 and p53 [48]. This again underscores the need for repeated PDT sessions with vigilant follow-up when using this field therapy for cancer prevention (see Table 5.3).

Table 5.3 Summary of the treatment approach for AK and BD in OTR

Pretreatment
Consider curettage or keratolytics
Preconditioning with 5FU cream, CO_2 laser, microneedling
Treatment
ALA or MAL-PDT
2 sessions, 1–2 weeks apart
Red light → deeper penetration
Cyclical q several months → prevention
Location: face, hands more amendable
Nonresponding lesions → biopsy

Conversely, the use of PDT for primary treatment of AK or BD is much more straightforward, with available data suggesting that at least two PDT sessions 1–2 weeks apart are enough to provide adequate clearance of AK or BD lesions for up to 3 months [14]. Importantly, several studies have also noted differences in therapeutic response rates depending on lesion location, with poorer responses often seen in the arms and hands compared to the scalp and face [24, 29]. For example, Piaserico et al. showed a significantly higher response rate of scalp/facial AKs treated with PDT compared to acral lesions (72 % vs 40 %, respectively) [24]. Others have noted similar trends with assessment of significance often limited by low study power [29]. Despite similar limitations in sample size, current studies on PDT in BCC have conversely shown no obvious difference in treatment response with relation to lesional site location [22, 32, 34]. Regardless of lesion type or location, however, any lesion not responding to PDT warrants biopsy.

5.2.6 Associated Risks

A theoretical risk of further immunosuppression surrounds the use of PDT in OTRs; however, scant data exists to substantiate this concern.

Matthews et al. have reported significant suppression of delayed-type hypersensitivity responses to tuberculin purified protein derivative (Mantoux reactions) in healthy control patients (Mantoux-positive volunteers) following treatment with either MAL-PDT or ALA-PDT [50]. Additionally, Nobbe et al. documented a case of HSV reactivation following PDT [51]. Beyond these limited cases, however, there is no compelling evidence that PDT has long-term deleterious effects on the immune system [14]. Nonetheless, Frost and colleagues have proposed that immunosuppression can be avoided by reducing the rate of irradiation while maintaining light doses during PDT [52].

Beyond fear of risking added immunosuppression, another common concern surrounding PDT in the OTR population is risk of organ damage, especially that of the transplant graft itself. An analysis of reported adverse events in 200+ OTRs undergoing PDT by Basset-Seguin and colleagues revealed no cases of reported graft damage [53].

In reality, pain is by far the most common, and limiting, adverse event associated with PDT. Pain most often occurs early during illumination with a minority of patients reporting pain, burning sensation, itching, and blisters shortly thereafter [29, 40]. Given the larger size, number, and involvement of lesions, pain is often significantly greater in the OTR population, especially in field cancerization areas such as the head and scalp [14, 54]. Several, well-studied, pain-relieving techniques are available to complement the delivery of PDT including use of cooling fans, intralesional anesthetics, nerve blocks, transcutaneous electrical nerve stimulation, and modified treatment delivery protocols [55]. Unfortunately, limited pretreatment predictors exist to help identify those patients who would benefit most from such interventions [54].

Earlier studies have shown that irradiance can affect pain threshold and high irradiance can also lead to oxygen depletion with high photosensitizer levels, which ultimately leads to inefficient treatments. A two-step irradiance approach was developed and studied in an open-label trial for BCC using ALA and the argon-pumped dye laser [55]. Lesions were first illuminated with a low irradiance until 90 % of the protoporphyrin IX was photobleached and then switched to a higher irradiance for a similar total light dose. Minimal patient discomfort was found with treatment outcomes similar to continuous irradiance data. In a follow-up prospective study with MAL and either argon laser or commercially available LED with a neutral density filter, the two-step irradiance approach findings were confirmed of little to no treatment-related pain and similar clinical outcomes [56].

Conclusions

PDT offers many advantages over conventional therapies ideal for the OTR population. As a noninvasive, office-based field therapy, it provides a convenient and repeatable treatment for large lesional areas, which complements the often widespread and numerous malignant and premalignant lesions common to the OTR population (Fig. 5.1). This convenience comes with added functional gain in that PDT has been shown be equally efficacious as conventional therapies with superior cosmetic outcomes and fewer reports of serious adverse events, such as life-threatening surgical infections, making it ideal for the underlying immunosuppression found in OTRs [29, 30, 33]. Indeed, PDT is especially useful for large widespread lesions in anatomically or cosmetically challenging areas where frequent and/or complicated surgeries may not be feasible. Additionally, PDT lacks the side effects common to chemotherapy and radiation therapies commonly used in oncology and, more importantly, remains immune to mechanisms of radio- and chemoresistance, making it an attractive treatment option for advanced disease as well [4].

Overall, the attractive side effect profile of PDT derives from the short duration and superficial nature of the treatment itself [1, 4]. Ironically, this strength also doubles as a limitation, as the highly localized nature of the therapy makes it ineffective against metastatic lesions, which are the most common cause of cancer-related mortality [4]. Despite this significant limitation, however, it is obvious that the strengths of PDT are abundant, with most well-suited for the OTR population. Most importantly, the advantages of PDT have translated into patient satisfaction, and, not surprisingly, evidence shows patients often prefer PDT over conventional therapies [57, 58].

References

1. Braathen LR, et al. Photodynamic therapy for skin field cancerization: an international consensus. International Society for Photodynamic Therapy in Dermatology. J Eur Acad Dermatol Venereol. 2012;26(9):1063–6.
2. Babilas P, et al. Photodynamic therapy in dermatology: state-of-the-art. Photodermatol Photoimmunol Photomed. 2010;26(3):118–32.
3. Sidoroff A, Thaler P. Taking treatment decisions in non-melanoma skin cancer – the place for topical photodynamic therapy (PDT). Photodiagnosis Photodyn Ther. 2010;7(1):24–32.
4. Agostinis P, et al. Photodynamic therapy of cancer: an update. CA Cancer J Clin. 2011;61(4):250–81.
5. Korbelik M. PDT-associated host response and its role in the therapy outcome. Lasers Surg Med. 2006;38(5): 500–8
6. Allison RR, Sibata CH. Oncologic photodynamic therapy photosensitizers: a clinical review. Photodiagnosis Photodyn Ther. 2010;7(2):61–75.
7. De Rosa FS, Bentley MV. Photodynamic therapy of skin cancers: sensitizers, clinical studies and future directives. Pharm Res. 2000;17(12):1447–55.
8. Plaetzer K, et al. Photophysics and photochemistry of photodynamic therapy: fundamental aspects. Lasers Med Sci. 2009;24(2):259–68.
9. Hamblin MR, Newman EL. On the mechanism of the tumour-localising effect in photodynamic therapy. J Photochem Photobiol B. 1994;23(1):3–8.
10. Brancaleon L, Moseley H. Laser and non-laser light sources for photodynamic therapy. Lasers Med Sci. 2002;17(3):173–86.
11. Euvrard S, et al. Comparative epidemiologic study of premalignant and malignant epithelial cutaneous lesions developing after kidney and heart transplantation. J Am Acad Dermatol. 1995;33(2 Pt 1):222–9.
12. Berg D, Otley CC. Skin cancer in organ transplant recipients: epidemiology, pathogenesis, and management. J Am Acad Dermatol. 2002;47(1):1–17; quiz 18–20.
13. Hartevelt MM, et al. Incidence of skin cancer after renal transplantation in The Netherlands. Transplantation. 1990;49(3):506–9.
14. Wlodek C, Ali FR, Lear JT. Use of photodynamic therapy for treatment of actinic keratoses in organ transplant recipients. Biomed Res Int. 2013;2013:349526.
15. Lindelof B, et al. Incidence of skin cancer in 5356 patients following organ transplantation. Br J Dermatol. 2000;143(3):513–9.
16. Stockfleth E, et al. Epithelial malignancies in organ transplant patients: clinical presentation and new methods of treatment. Recent Results Cancer Res. 2002;160:251–8.
17. Webb MC, et al. Skin tumours posttransplantation: a retrospective analysis of 28 years' experience at a single centre. Transplant Proc. 1997;29(1–2):828–30.
18. Adamson R, et al. High incidence and clinical course of aggressive skin cancer in heart transplant patients: a single-center study. Transplant Proc. 1998;30(4):1124–6.
19. Martinez JC, et al. Defining the clinical course of metastatic skin cancer in organ transplant recipients: a multicenter collaborative study. Arch Dermatol. 2003; 139(3):301–6.
20. Euvrard S, et al. Subsequent skin cancers in kidney and heart transplant recipients after the first squamous cell carcinoma. Transplantation. 2006;81(8):1093–100.
21. Wisgerhof HC, et al. Subsequent squamous- and basal-cell carcinomas in kidney-transplant recipients after the first skin cancer: cumulative incidence and risk factors. Transplantation. 2010;89(10):1231–8.
22. Schleier P, et al. Photodynamic therapy of virus-associated epithelial tumours of the face in organ transplant recipients. J Cancer Res Clin Oncol. 2004; 130(5):279–84.
23. Dragieva G, et al. A randomized controlled clinical trial of topical photodynamic therapy with methyl aminolaevulinate in the treatment of actinic keratoses in transplant recipients. Br J Dermatol. 2004;151(1): 196–200.
24. Piaserico S, et al. Topical photodynamic therapy of actinic keratosis in renal transplant recipients. Transplant Proc. 2007;39(6):1847–50.
25. Wennberg AM, et al. Photodynamic therapy with methyl aminolevulinate for prevention of new skin lesions in transplant recipients: a randomized study. Transplantation. 2008;86(3):423–9.
26. Hasson A, et al. Topical photodynamic therapy with methylaminolevulinate for the treatment of actinic keratosis and reduction of photodamage in organ transplant recipients: a case-series of 16 patients. Indian J Dermatol Venereol Leprol. 2012;78(4):448–53.
27. Bencini PL, et al. Application of photodynamic therapy combined with pre-illumination microneedling in the treatment of actinic keratosis in organ transplant recipients. Br J Dermatol. 2012;167(5):1193–4.
28. Helsing P, et al. Intensified fractional CO2 laser-assisted photodynamic therapy vs. laser alone for organ transplant recipients with multiple actinic keratoses and wart-like lesions: a randomized half-side comparative trial on dorsal hands. Br J Dermatol. 2013;169(5):1087–92.
29. Dragieva G, et al. Topical photodynamic therapy in the treatment of actinic keratoses and Bowen's disease in transplant recipients. Transplantation. 2004;77(1):115–21.
30. Perrett CM, et al. Treatment of post-transplant premalignant skin disease: a randomized intrapatient comparative study of 5-fluorouracil cream and topical photodynamic therapy. Br J Dermatol. 2007;156(2): 320–8.

31. Perrett CM, et al. Treatment of basal cell carcinoma with topical methylaminolaevulinate photodynamic therapy in an organ-transplant recipient. Clin Exp Dermatol. 2006;31(1):146–7.
32. Guleng GE, Helsing P. Photodynamic therapy for basal cell carcinomas in organ-transplant recipients. Clin Exp Dermatol. 2012;37(4):367–9.
33. Szeimies RM, et al. Photodynamic therapy using topical methyl 5-aminolevulinate compared with cryotherapy for actinic keratosis: a prospective, randomized study. J Am Acad Dermatol. 2002;47(2):258–62.
34. Collier NJ, Ali FR, Lear JT. Efficacy of photodynamic therapy for treatment of basal cell carcinoma in organ transplant recipients. Lasers Med Sci 2013, Oct 15. Epub ahead of print.
35. Maytin EV, et al. Clinical studies of combined photodynamic therapy using 5-fluorouracil and methyl-aminolevulinate in patients at high risk for squamous cell carcinoma. In: Optical methods for tumor treatment and detection: mechanisms and techniques in photodynamic therapy XXII. San Francisco: SPIE Proceedings; 2013.
36. Togsverd-Bo K, et al. Intensified photodynamic therapy of actinic keratoses with fractional CO2 laser: a randomized clinical trial. Br J Dermatol. 2012;166(6):1262–9.
37. Clementoni MT, B-Roscher M, Munavalli GS. Photodynamic photorejuvenation of the face with a combination of microneedling, red light, and broadband pulsed light. Lasers Surg Med. 2010;42(2):150–9.
38. Torezan L, et al. A pilot split-face study comparing conventional methyl aminolevulinate-photodynamic therapy (PDT) with microneedling-assisted PDT on actinically damaged skin. Dermatol Surg. 2013;39(8): 1197–201.
39. Wulf HC, et al. Topical photodynamic therapy for prevention of new skin lesions in renal transplant recipients. Acta Derm Venereol. 2006;86(1):25–8.
40. de Graaf YG, et al. Photodynamic therapy does not prevent cutaneous squamous-cell carcinoma in organ-transplant recipients: results of a randomized-controlled trial. J Invest Dermatol. 2006;126(3):569–74.
41. Willey A, Mehta S, Lee PK. Reduction in the incidence of squamous cell carcinoma in solid organ transplant recipients treated with cyclic photodynamic therapy. Dermatol Surg. 2010;36(5):652–8.
42. Stender IM, et al. Photodynamic therapy with topical delta-aminolevulinic acid delays UV photocarcinogenesis in hairless mice. Photochem Photobiol. 1997;66(4):493–6.
43. Liu Y, Viau G, Bissonnette R. Multiple large-surface photodynamic therapy sessions with topical or systemic aminolevulinic acid and blue light in UV-exposed hairless mice. J Cutan Med Surg. 2004;8(2):131–9.
44. Sharfaei S, et al. Weekly topical application of methyl aminolevulinate followed by light exposure delays the appearance of UV-induced skin tumours in mice. Arch Dermatol Res. 2002;294(5):237–42.
45. Caty V, et al. Multiple large surface photodynamic therapy sessions with topical methylaminolaevulinate in PTCH heterozygous mice. Br J Dermatol. 2006; 154(4):740–2.
46. Apalla Z, et al. Skin cancer: preventive photodynamic therapy in patients with face and scalp cancerization. A randomized placebo-controlled study. Br J Dermatol. 2010;162(1):171–5.
47. Steinbauer JM, et al. Topical photodynamic therapy with porphyrin precursors – assessment of treatment-associated pain in a retrospective study. Photochem Photobiol Sci. 2009;8(8):1111–6.
48. Bagazgoitia L, et al. Photodynamic therapy reduces the histological features of actinic damage and the expression of early oncogenic markers. Br J Dermatol. 2011;165(1):144–51.
49. Szeimies RM, et al. Clinical, histopathological and immunohistochemical assessment of human skin field cancerization before and after photodynamic therapy. Br J Dermatol. 2012;167(1):150–9.
50. Matthews YJ, Damian DL. Topical photodynamic therapy is immunosuppressive in humans. Br J Dermatol. 2010;162(3):637–41.
51. Nobbe S, et al. Herpes simplex virus reactivation as a complication of photodynamic therapy. Photodermatol Photoimmunol Photomed. 2011;27(1):51–2.
52. Frost GA, Halliday GM, Damian DL. Photodynamic therapy-induced immunosuppression in humans is prevented by reducing the rate of light delivery. J Invest Dermatol. 2011;131(4):962–8.
53. Basset-Seguin N, et al. Photodynamic therapy for actinic keratosis in organ transplant patients. J Eur Acad Dermatol Venereol. 2013;27(1):57–66.
54. Arits AH, et al. Pain during topical photodynamic therapy: uncomfortable and unpredictable. J Eur Acad Dermatol Venereol. 2010;24(12):1452–7.
55. Zeitouni NC, et al. A retrospective review of pain control by a two-step irradiance schedule during topical ALA-photodynamic therapy of non-melanoma skin cancer. Lasers Surg Med. 2013;45(2):89–94.
56. Zeitouni NC, et al. A prospective study of pain control by a 2-step irradiance schedule during topical photodynamic therapy of nonmelanoma skin cancer. Dermatol surg vol. 2014;40(12):1390–94.
57. Braathen LR, et al. Guidelines on the use of photodynamic therapy for nonmelanoma skin cancer: an international consensus. International Society for Photodynamic Therapy in Dermatology, 2005. J Am Acad Dermatol. 2007;56(1):125–43.
58. Weston A, Fitzgerald P. Discrete choice experiment to derive willingness to pay for methyl aminolevulinate photodynamic therapy versus simple excision surgery in basal cell carcinoma. Pharmacoeconomics. 2004; 22(18):1195–208.

6 Update on Staging, Definition, and Chemoprevention of "High-Risk Squamous Cell Carcinoma" in Organ Transplant Recipients

Cameron Chesnut, Ashley G. Rubin, Stephanie Jeanne Martin, Joseph Diehl, and Teresa Soriano

Contents

C. Chesnut, MD
Internal Medicine, Dermatologic Surgery, University of Washington School of Medicine, Spokane, WA, USA
e-mail: cameronchesnut@gmail.com

A.G. Rubin, MD
Division of Dermatology, Department of Medicine, University of California, San Diego, San Diego, CA, USA
e-mail: Ashley.gale.rubin@gmail.com

S.J. Martin, MD
Division of Dermatology, UCLA, Los Angeles, CA, USA
e-mail: sjmartin@mednet.ucla.edu

J. Diehl, MD
Division of Dermatology, Department of Medicine, UCLA, Los Angeles, CA, USA
e-mail: jdiehl@mednet.ucla.edu

T. Soriano, MD (✉)
Department of Medicine/Dermatology, UCLA School of Medicine, Los Angeles, CA, USA
e-mail: tsoriano@mednet.ucla.edu

In the general population, most cutaneous squamous cell carcinomas (SCC) are cured with surgical excision or destruction. However, according to two large cohort studies, 3.7–4 % of those cutaneous SCC patients develop metastases or unresectable local recurrence [1, 2], and a group of those with such advanced tumors ultimately die of the disease. When compared to the general population, organ transplant recipients (OTRs) have a 65- to 250-fold increased risk of developing cutaneous SCC [3], making staging, prognosis, and treatment determinations especially important, all the while lacking full clarity in the literature. With this increased risk of SCC development in addition to higher tumor burden, more aggressive cutaneous carcinomas [4–8], and increased risk of metastasis and skin cancer-related mortality [8, 4, 5, 7], OTRs also represent a desirable target for additional preventive measures in the form of chemoprevention.

F. Zwald, M.D. Brown (eds.), *Advances in Transplant Dermatology: Clinical and Practical Implications*, DOI 10.1007/978-3-319-12445-2_6,

6.1 Staging of Cutaneous Squamous Cell Carcinoma

In 2010, the American Joint Committee on Cancer (AJCC) published the 7th edition of the staging system for cutaneous squamous cell carcinomas. There were a few revisions of the new staging system, namely, separating carcinomas of the eyelid from other skin surfaces. The staging system for non-eyelid skin cancers is primarily designed for squamous cell carcinomas; however, the staging system for carcinoma of the eyelid addresses various histologic types of carcinomas (including but not limited to squamous cell carcinoma) [9].

The staging of cutaneous squamous cell carcinoma, excluding carcinoma of the eyelid, is separated into four stages. These four stages are determined by the primary tumor (T), lymph node involvement (N), and distant metastases (M). Patients with a primary cutaneous squamous cell carcinoma with no evidence of regional or distant metastases, based on either clinical, radiologic, or pathologic evidence, are divided into either stage 1 or stage 2. Stage 1 tumors are clinically measured to be 2 cm or less in size. Stage 2 tumors are clinically measured to be greater than 2 cm in size. In instances where there is clinical concern regarding the extension of the tumor into bone, and radiologic evaluation has been performed, and there is no evidence of deeper extension, these data may be included to support the stage 1 versus stage 2 designation. However, tumors that are clinically measured to be 2 cm or less in size, thus qualifying for stage 1 designation, can be upstaged to stage 2 if they contain two or more high-risk features. The introduction of a list of high-risk clinical and histologic features that can modify the T (tumor size) designation is one of the most significant changes to the new staging system. These high-risk features include a tumor thickness of more than 2 mm, a Clark level of IV or more, location on the external ear or non-glabrous lip, perineural invasion, bone involvement, and poor tumor differentiation [9].

Stage 3 is classified as those tumors with either of the following: clinical, histologic, or radiologic evidence of one involved lymph node measuring 3 cm or less in size or tumor extension into bone, namely, the maxilla, mandible, orbit, or temporal bone. Stage 4 is classified if any of the following criteria are met: a tumor with direct or perineural invasion of the skull base or axial skeleton, two or more involved lymph nodes, single or multiple involved lymph nodes measuring more than 3 cm in size, or distant metastases (Tables 6.1 and 6.2) [9].

Table 6.1 The AJCC TNM classification of cutaneous SCC (non-eyelid)

Tx	Primary tumor cannot be assessed
T0	No evidence of primary tumor
Tis	Carcinoma in situ
T1	Tumor ≥2 cm in greatest dimension with <2 high-risk features[a]
T2	Tumor >2 cm in greatest dimension
	or
	Tumor of any size with ≥2 high-risk features[a]
T3	Tumor with invasion of maxilla, mandible, orbit, or temporal bone
T4	Tumor with invasion of skeleton (axial or appendicular) or perineural invasion of skull base
Nx	Regional lymph nodes cannot be assessed
N0	No regional lymph node metastases
N1	Metastasis in a single ipsilateral lymph node, ≤3 cm in greatest dimension
N2a	Metastasis in a single ipsilateral lymph node, >3 cm but ≤6 cm in greatest dimension
N2b	Metastasis in multiple ipsilateral lymph nodes ≤6 cm in greatest dimension
N2c	Metastasis in bilateral or contralateral lymph nodes, ≤6 cm in greatest dimension
N3	Metastasis in a lymph node, >6 cm in greatest dimension
M0	No distant metastases
M1	Distant metastases

[a]High-risk features for primary tumor (T) staging: >2 mm thickness (Breslow thickness), Clark level ≥IV, perineural invasion, primary site of the ear, primary site of the hair-bearing lip, poorly differentiated or undifferentiated

6.1.1 Eyelid Carcinomas

As previously mentioned, the revised AJCC staging separates eyelid carcinomas from other cutaneous squamous cell carcinomas. The TNM classification is used to stage all cell types of

Table 6.2 Staging for cutaneous squamous cell carcinomas (non-eyelid)

Stage	T	N	M
0	Tis	N0	M0
1	T1	N0	M0
2	T2	N0	M0
3	T3	N0	M0
	T1	N1	M0
	T2	N1	M0
	T3	N1	M0
4	T1	N2	M0
	T2	N2	M0
	T3	N2	M0
	Any T	N3	M0
	T4	Any N	M0
	Any T	Any N	M1

Table 6.3 Staging for eyelid carcinomas (including squamous cell carcinomas)

Stage	T	N	M
0	Tis	N0	M0
1A	T1	N0	M0
1B	T2a	N0	M0
1C	T2b	N0	M0
2	T3a	N0	M0
3A	T3b	N0	M0
3B	Any T	N1	M0
3C	T4	Any N	M0
4	Any T	Any N	M1

eyelid carcinomas, including squamous cell carcinoma. The Tx, T0, and Tis is staged similarly as for non-eyelid skin. The staging differences for eyelid skin becomes a factor for the T1 designation and higher. T1 applies to a tumor that is 5 mm or less in greatest dimension AND does not invade the tarsal plate or eyelid margin. T2a applies to a tumor that is greater than 5 mm but not greater than 10 mm in greatest dimension *OR* any tumor that invades the tarsal plate or eyelid margin. T2b applies to a tumor that is greater than 10 mm but not greater than 20 mm in greatest dimension *OR* involves the full thickness eyelid. T3a designation is applied to a tumor that meets any of the following criteria: greater than 20 mm in greatest dimension, *OR* any tumor that invades adjacent ocular or orbital structures, *OR* a tumor of any size that demonstrates perineural invasion. T3b designation is applied to a tumor that requires enucleation for complete tumor resection, exenteration, or bone resection. T4 applies to a tumor that is not resectable due to extensive invasion of either ocular, orbital, and craniofacial structures or the brain. The regional lymph node designation of Nx (regional lymph nodes cannot be assessed) is the same as for non-eyelid skin. cN0 applies to no regional lymph node metastasis based upon clinical evaluation or imaging, and pN0 applies to no regional lymph node metastasis based upon lymph node biopsy. N1 applies to regional lymph node metastasis. Distant metastasis criteria are the same for eyelid squamous cell carcinomas as non-eyelid cutaneous squamous cell carcinomas (Table 6.3) [10].

6.1.2 Application of Updated Staging to Transplant Patients

The revised staging system is more clearly defined than previous staging, including separation of eyelid squamous cell carcinomas from non-eyelid cutaneous squamous cell carcinomas and incorporation of high-risk features. However, there is concern that the current staging system requires additional updates. There have been several proposed revisions to the current staging system with concern that the current criteria defining high-risk cutaneous squamous cell carcinomas are not sufficiently accurate and thus may reduce survival and hinder management of the disease according to risk.

The first validation study of the new AJCC T staging system by using patient outcome data showed that the bulk of poor outcomes (83 % of nodal metastases and 92 % of disease-specific deaths) occurred in AJCC T2 tumors. Investigators at Brigham and Women's Hospital proposed an alternate T staging system with the aim of better stratifying the stage T2 group into low-risk T2a and high-risk T2b categories. Four risk factors were found to be statistically independent prognostic factors, including poor differentiation, perineural invasion, tumor diameter ≥2 cm, and invasion beyond subcutaneous fat and were thus incorporated in the alternative staging with 0 factors indicating T1; 1 factor indicating T2a;

Table 6.4 Proposed alternative tumor staging system for SCC

Alternative tumor staging system for cutaneous SCC[a]	
Primary tumor	Criteria[b]
T0	In situ squamous cell carcinoma
T1	0 risk factors
T2a	1 risk factor
T2b	2–3 risk factors
T3	4 risk factors or bone invasion

[a]Adapted from Jambusaria-Pahlajani et al. [11]
[b]Risk factors include tumor diameter of 2 cm or greater, poorly differentiated histological characteristics, perineural invasion, and tumor invasion beyond the subcutaneous fat (excluding bone invasion, which automatically upgrades the tumor to alternative stage T3)

2–3 factors, T2b; and 4 factors or bone invasion, T3. Stages T2a and T2b significantly differed in incidences of all 4 end points. The high-risk T2b group contained a minority of the patients (19 % of the cohort) but the majority of poor outcomes (72 % nodal metastases and 83 % of disease-specific deaths). Therefore, this proposed staging system may offer improved outcome similarity within stages as well as worsening outcome with increasing stage [11] (Table 6.4).

This proposed staging system was further validated in a subsequent study, comparing Brigham and Women's Hospital (BWH) tumor staging system with the AJCC staging system. The BWH staging system divides AJCC T2 tumors into two separate groups, a large low-risk T2a group and a smaller high-risk T2b group, and collapses AJCC T3/T4 (bone invasion tumors) into a single BWH T3 group, which also includes rare high-risk tumors with all four risk factors but no bone invasion. BWH T2b and T3 together account for a small fraction (5 %) of cutaneous squamous cell carcinomas but a large majority of local recurrences, nodal metastases, and disease-related deaths (47 %, 70 %, and 83 %, respectively). Conversely, BWH T2b and T3 tumors had a 21 % (95 % CI, 14–31 %) and 67 % (95 % CI, 30–90 %) risk of nodal metastases, respectively [12]. Therefore, cumulative incidences of poor outcomes were low for BWH low-stage (T1/T2a) tumors and higher for high-stage (T2b/T3) tumors, thus further validating the earlier study of an alternative staging system.

It has also been suggested that while anatomic location and lack of perineural invasion are good prognostic predictors, the subjectivity of tumor differentiation and the importance of the Clark level are not as well defined. Furthermore the differentiation between low-risk and high-risk cutaneous squamous cell carcinomas is currently defined by the cutoff of 2 mm for the depth of tumor invasion. It has been suggested that this is a poor marker given that a significant number of cutaneous SCCs are thicker than 2 mm. Thus, the current depth cutoff allows for higher sensitivity but decreased specificity in terms of predicting risk [13].

Additionally, although the new AJCC staging system includes several "high-risk" factors, there are several other factors that have been proposed to be included in the staging system. Immunosuppression has been demonstrated to negatively contribute to prognosis and thus has been proposed to be reflected in the staging system. The current TNM criteria exclude clinical risk factors in staging, including immunosuppression [14].

Furthermore, recurrent cutaneous squamous cell carcinomas have been shown to be associated with a higher rate of lymph node metastases. A comparative analysis of lymph node metastasis in recurrent versus primary cutaneous squamous cell carcinomas was 15 % and 2 %, respectively ($P<.001$) [15]. Cutaneous squamous cell carcinoma recurrence has also been correlated to tumor size, with larger tumors associated with a significantly higher rate of recurrence. Finally, recurrent lesions have been associated with a higher rate of perineural invasion, lymphovascular invasion, and subcutaneous tissue invasion [16]. As tumor recurrence has been demonstrated to be an important risk factor in cutaneous squamous cell carcinoma, it has been proposed that tumor recurrence should be included in the high-risk classification [15].

Other factors that have been proposed as possible prognostic factors in cutaneous squamous cell carcinoma are peritumoral actinic keratoses, various Clark levels, desmoplasia, and Ki67 expression [1, 17]. The true prognostic value of these factors still needs to be further elucidated by additional studies.

6.2 Definition of High-Risk Cutaneous Squamous Cell Carcinoma

High-risk cutaneous SCCs are those tumors associated with a high risk of subclinical metastasis and thus adverse events including local recurrence, nodal metastases, and disease-specific death [13]. As previously mentioned, immunosuppression adversely affects outcomes in transplant patients with SCC, and lack of sufficient prospective data in these patients makes establishing high-risk criteria difficult [13, 14]. Risk factors often occur together, and studies with sufficient subjects to calculate outcomes with multivariate (as opposed to univariate) modeling to control for this coexistence are limited [2]. Proposed "high-risk" factors will be discussed independently, as several consensus guidelines have been published but with differing definitions [18], and criticism that important factors are excluded, or are overly sensitive as to include many low-risk tumors [13]. With no universally accepted standard definition of high-risk features, these are often defined on a study-by-study basis, with some using the terms "high risk" and "very high risk." [19]. Immunosuppression itself is considered high risk in some guidelines (National Comprehensive Cancer Network, NCCN) but not others (American Joint Committee on Cancer, AJCC). As always, prospective multicenter studies looking into transplant patients in particular are needed to better define "high risk" in an already high-risk population. Clinical and histologic factors are the most studied indicators of high risk, but recent work on molecular factors will likely become relevant with more research.

6.2.1 Immunosuppression After Transplantation

Cutaneous SCC is seen in over one quarter of heart and lung transplant patients within 5 years [20]. Immunosuppression for longer periods is associated with progressively higher incidence of SCC, with 45 % at 11 years and 70 % at 20 years in kidney and heart transplant patients [5]. Mortality, metastases, and recurrences are all increased in transplant patients, with heart transplant recipients most affected and then lung, kidney, and finally liver recipients [13]. In a prospective study, immunosuppression was found to have a hazard ratio of 4.32 for the development of metastases [1], while observation of patients treated for nodal metastases from head and neck cutaneous SCC saw 39 % of immunosuppressed patients experienced local recurrence, versus only 15 % of the immunocompetent patients [21]. Similarly, Martinez et al. observed a 5 % mortality from SCC in transplant patients compared to 1 % in immunocompetent patients [22].

Immunosuppression is included in high-risk criteria in the NCCN guidelines, but not the AJCC, as clinical risk factors are precluded from the staging system, although it recommended that such information be collected and used in data study [18]. Immunosuppression is a major criterion in the high-risk definition proposed by Martorell [13].

Separate from iatrogenic immunosuppression, human immunodeficiency virus (HIV) infection portends worse prognosis, regardless of CD4+ T cell counts, with 5 of 10 HIV patients with high-risk SCC dying within 7 years in a small study [23], suggesting another instance in which immune system alteration affects the course of SCC.

6.2.2 Tumor Diameter

Clinical tumor diameter of 2.0 cm or greater is considered a high-risk feature of cutaneous SCC in the AJCC and NCCN guidelines and supported by many studies [5, 18, 20, 22, 24]. Metastatic rates of these larger SCC were triple those less than 2.0 cm (30 % vs 9 %) [25], while a retrospective cohort with multivariate analysis found a 5.6-fold subhazard ratio (SHR) of local recurrence, 7.0-fold SHR for metastases, and 15.9-fold SHR for disease-specific death [2]. A retrospective cohort evaluation of the AJCC guidelines detected a 4.2 SHR for local recurrence and 3.7 SHR for disease-specific death [11]. Some studies have attempted to identify further size increases with adverse outcomes but are too limited to be included at this time [16, 18].

6.2.3 Tumor Location

The AJCC identifies only the non-glabrous lip and ear as high-risk sites [9, 18], while the NCCN guidelines identify the "mask areas" of the face (central face, eyelids, eyebrows, nose, lips, chin, mandible, ears and periorbital and pre-/postauricular areas) and genitals, hands, and feet as high risk [24]. The external ear and non-glabrous lip have some of the highest incidence of metastases from SCC (20–30 %) [21, 13], although in a multivariate analysis of over 1,800 patients, it was found that while the ear and temple had a hazard ratio of 3.8 for metastases and 6.9 for disease-specific death (lip was not higher than any other head or neck sites), anogenital SCCs had an HR of 4.1 for metastases and 23.7 for disease-specific death [2]. In the high-risk definition proposed by Martorell, lip, anogenital, and external ear are all considered major criteria [13]. A prospective study by Brantsch of 615 patients found only the ear to be associated with increased metastatic risk (hazard ratio 3.61) [1]. Specific to transplant populations, a study of heart and lung transplant recipients did not detect a higher risk for recurrence or metastasis on the lip or ear, though only 41 patients with 225 SCC were included [20].

Additionally, SCCs occurring at sites of previous skin injury – including scars, chronic ulcers, and sites of radiation dermatitis – have increased metastatic risk [13] and are considered high-risk criteria in the NCCN guidelines [24]. Such locations are considered minor criteria in the high-risk definition proposed by Martorell [13].

6.2.4 Tumor Recurrence

Recurrent tumors are associated with worse prognosis, with previously mentioned metastatic rates of 15 % in recurrent SCC and 2 % in primary SCC of the lip in one study [26] and metastatic rates of 32 % and 45 % for recurrent SCC of lip and ear, respectively, in another [25]. Recurrent SCC is thus considered high risk in the NCCN guidelines [24] and minor criteria in the Martonell high-risk definition. Tumor recurrence is not included in the AJCC staging criteria [18].

6.2.5 Depth of Invasion

Both the AJCC and NCCN guidelines consider tumors with thickness of 2 mm or more, or depth of invasion to the reticular dermis/Clark level IV, as high-risk tumors [18, 24]. Many studies have shown that both are important prognostically in SCC [1, 17, 18, 25, 27, 28]. In one study, 325 lip SCCs less than 2 mm in thickness did not have a single metastasis, while those of 6 mm or more had a metastatic rate of 16 %. In the middle group, of 2.1–5.9 mm tumor thickness, 4 % had metastases [1]. Invasion of subcutaneous fat was associated with 4.1 % metastatic rate, while invasion of deeper tissues (muscle, bone) was 12.5 % [29]. Similarly, multivariate analysis of over 1,832 tumors found that depth of invasion beyond subcutaneous fat had a SHR of 7.2 for local recurrence compared to invasion of only the dermis or subcutaneous fat and SHR of disease-specific death of 13.0 [2]. A confirmatory retrospective application of AJCC staging guidelines found an identical SHR for depth of invasion beyond fat [11]; however, analysis of the 2 mm depth/ Clark level IV was not done. Clearly, invasion beyond the cuticular structures creates a high-risk tumor, and recent studies tend to use extension beyond fat, rather than Clark level IV or 2 mm depth, as the significant depth [2, 11, 19, 20]. Others suggest using 4 mm as a less sensitive, but more specific indicator of high risk [13]. Unfortunately, analysis of AJCC staging guidelines in heart and lung transplant patients with SCC did not include any tumors with invasion beyond the dermis, and which high-risk factors were used to meet staging criteria were not mentioned, so application of these important high-risk factors in the ideal patient population was not performed [20].

6.2.6 Tumor Differentiation and Histologic Subtype

The AJCC guidelines include poorly differentiated tumors as high risk [9], while the NCCN guidelines include moderately and poorly differentiated SCC. Although well-differentiated SCC can still cause advanced disease, poorly differentiated SCC had a 2.9-fold risk of death compared to well-differentiated SCC [30]. Two studies found consistent rates of metastasis of 4–5 % for well-differentiated tumors but 17–44 % for poorly differentiated tumors [25, 30]. In the largest retrospective multivariate study, moderately differentiated SCCs were grouped with the well-differentiated tumors (as in the AJCC classification), thus isolating the poorly differentiated SCC for comparison, which had SHRs of 3.3, 6.1, and 6.7 for recurrence, nodal metastasis, and disease-specific death, respectively [2].

Several histologic subtypes of SCC (adenoid, acantholytic, adenosquamous with mucin production, and desmoplastic) are also included in the NCCN high-risk category [24], as well as a revised high-risk classification proposed by Martorell et al. [13]. A large prospective study of 615 patients found desmoplasia associated with a risk of local recurrence of 16 times those of non-desmoplastic histology [1].

6.2.7 Perineural Invasion

Perineural invasion, whether macro- or microscopic, was seen in 5.9 % of SCC undergoing Mohs micrographic surgery in one study [31], but estimates range from 5 to 10 % [13]. In SCC of the face, perineural invasion is associated with increased local (35 % vs 15 %, $p<0.005$) and distant metastasis (15 % vs 3.3 %, $P<0.005$) and reduced survival [13, 32]. It is typically found in association with other high-risk factors, including larger tumors, poor differentiation (see above), recurrences, and location on the face [33]. In one study, the thickness of the nerves involved was seen as important. Tumors involving nerves less than 0.1 mm in diameter had 0 % disease-specific death versus 32 % in tumors involving nerves greater than 0.1 mm ($P=0.003$) [34]. In another retrospective cohort of 114 tumors with perineural invasion, only one local recurrence occurred with perineural invasion of small (<0.1 mm diameter) nerves in the absence of other risk factors. Larger involved nerves were more likely to be associated with other high-risk factors and adverse events [35]. However, nerve diameter is not currently considered in any guidelines [9, 24]. Clinical neurologic symptoms indicative of perineural invasion (tingling, pain, formication) are considered a high-risk factor in NCCN guidelines, irrespective of histologic or radiologic evidence of invasion [24].

6.2.8 Vascular Involvement

The NCCN guidelines consider vascular involvement a high-risk factor [24], while the AJCC guidelines do not. One study found vascular invasion to have an odds ratio of metastasis of 7.54 in multivariate analysis [36], and though its acceptance has been challenged [30], lymphovascular invasion has been included as minor criteria in a recent definition of high-risk SCC [13].

6.2.9 Molecular Markers

Although most cases of metastatic SCC have at least one high-risk feature, 20–30 % do not, indicating unknown risk factors exist, and molecular changes may be responsible [13]. Recent research has emerged showing strong D2-40 staining of podoplanin, a protein important in cell migration, motility, and associated with lymphatic invasion, may be a significant predictor of lymphatic metastasis, having a 6.1 odds ratio compared to low-intensity expression of D2-40 [37]. Epidermal growth factor receptor overexpression [38], p16 expression, and CKS1B gene amplification may prove useful to predicting tumor behavior and deepen our understanding of that behavior as well [13].

6.3 Chemoprevention

According to the American Cancer Society, many of the millions of skin cancers diagnosed annually are preventable [39]. In immunosuppressed OTRs, reducing morbidity from increased tumor burden and mortality from high-risk squamous cell carcinomas can be challenging. The basic idea of chemoprevention hinges upon the stepwise progression of carcinogenesis and the understanding that there are many steps between sun exposure and the development of a skin cancer [6, 40–42]. Chemoprevention differs from standard preventative strategies. Standard prevention is always necessary, especially in OTRs, and it includes various sun protection behaviors, clothing, sunscreen, and education [43]. Conversely, chemoprevention is defined as the use of natural, synthetic, or biologic agents to reverse, suppress, or prevent the stepwise carcinogenic progression [7, 42, 44]. Chemopreventive agents should be both effective and safe, causing minimal toxicity to normal cells [6, 44]. Chemoprevention is indicated in patients who are at a high risk for the development of many skin cancers or metastases; thus, OTRs automatically fit this indication [45]. Although the risk of cutaneous carcinoma development varies based on the type of organ transplant, OTRs remain the major target for chemoprevention [44, 46, 47]. When determining if a patient should be placed on a chemopreventive agent, several factors may be considered: the age of the individual at transplantation, prior history of sun exposure and skin cancers, the number of new skin cancers the patient is developing per year, the level of immunosuppression, and the patient's skin phototype [48–50].

6.3.1 Retinoids

Retinoids are similar to vitamin A either functionally or structurally and may be synthetically produced or occur naturally. All retinoids influence various genes through their action on retinoic acid and retinoid X receptors. Retinoids influence signal transduction, extracellular adhesion molecules, and expression of growth factors, in turn affecting cell proliferation, differentiation, and apoptosis. Taken together, these effects have been shown to prevent cancer development [51–57].

Several studies have explored the efficacy of retinoids as chemopreventive agents [45, 58–68]. Peck et al. conducted some of the first studies on oral retinoids as potential chemopreventives [59]. He demonstrated a reduction of skin cancers in five patients with xeroderma pigmentosum during a 2-year treatment period with systemic retinoids. Unfortunately, on discontinuation of the systemic treatment, the frequency of skin cancer in the posttreatment year increased to 8.5-fold over that of the treatment period [59]. The Southwest Skin Cancer Prevention Study of 1997 assessed the effects of oral retinoids in moderate and high-risk subjects [58]. Following 5 years of daily dosing with 25,000 IU of retinol or placebo, a significantly lower risk of developing a first new SCC was demonstrated in the moderate-risk treatment group – defined as having a history of more than 10 actinic keratoses and at most two nonmelanoma skin cancers (NMSCs) [58]. There was no difference in time to development of the first SCC in the high-risk group – defined as patients with four or more previous NMSCs [58]. Subsequently, Nijsten and colleagues found that in patients with psoriasis who had been previously treated with psoralen and ultraviolet light A (PUVA), systemic retinoids reduced SCC risk by 30 % but not basal cell carcinoma (BCC) risk [64].

The use of oral retinoids has also been studied in OTRs. A randomized control trial in renal transplant patients showed that those treated with oral acitretin 30 mg/day had significantly lower numbers of new tumors and total tumors (the presence of both SCCs and BCCs was evaluated) [60]. The chemopreventive effect was more pronounced in OTRs who had a previous history of skin cancer [60]. An additional study in renal transplant patients demonstrated that for those treated with acitretin (at a dose of 0.3 mg/kg/day), there was not only a dramatically decreased number of NMSCs, but also the chemopreventive effect was sustained over a 4-year period [62]. Moreover, a prospective, randomized crossover trial, administering acitretin at 25 mg daily, resulted in a significant decrease in SCCs and BCCs in renal transplant patients [65]. Similarly, another retrospective study in OTRs found a reduction in the development of cutaneous SCCs for those treated with acitretin or etretinate [67]. A study by de Sevaux et al. failed to demonstrate a reduction in SCC incidence with two different doses of acitretin; it has been postulated that this negative result was due to the short study period and the lack of a placebo group for comparison [6, 66]. There are currently ongoing randomized controlled trials assessing the chemopreventive efficacy of acitretin in OTRs. Etretinate, which is no longer available for patient use, was also found to be effective (at a dose of 0.3 mg/kg/day) in reducing the occurrence of skin cancer in renal transplant patients, but the positive benefit was only significant during the first 6 months of therapy [68].

Chemoprevention with oral retinoids should be considered when the benefits outweigh the risks of administration and used in conjunction with standard prevention strategies while carefully monitoring for side effects [6]. For specific administration guidelines, Soltani-Arabshahi et al. recommend to start with 10 mg of acitretin every other day and, while monitoring for side effects and incidence of NMSCs, and increase the dose by 10–20 mg per day every 2–4 weeks with a target dose of 15–25 mg per day [44]. Although acitretin is generally used as a first-line agent with more literature assessing long-term effects in OTRs, isotretinoin has been proven as a chemopreventive agent as well and would be the preferred agent in women of childbearing age based on its shorter half-life. If using isotretinoin, this group recommends to start with 0.25 mg/kg every other day and increase by 0.125–0.25 mg/kg per day if tolerable with a goal of 0.5 mg/kg / day [44]. The chemopreventive effect begins within months of administration of the oral agent, but the benefit ceases within months of discontinuation and both efficacy and side effects are dose dependent [6, 41, 44]. Due to this observed rebound effect with discontinuation, patients should be maintained on systemic retinoids for continued prevention. Side effects are variable depending on the dose and may include mucocutaneous reactions, hyperlipidemia, abnormalities in liver function tests, skeletal changes, increased intracranial pressure, and teratogenic effects [44]. As OTRs are commonly on other medications that can have similar adverse effects, such as elevations of liver enzymes and triglycerides, close monitoring with laboratory tests is essential particularly upon initiation and increase in dosages of oral retinoids.

6.3.2 Topical Retinoids

Topical retinoids have been used off-label in attempts to prevent actinic keratoses (AKs) and NMSCs [69]. Although some positive data exist, routine use is not generally supported [70–72]. Smit et al. failed to note a reduction in AKs in renal transplant patients who were treated with twice daily tretinoin cream alone or in combination with calcipotriol cream, albeit only over a 6-week period [72]. Weinstock and colleagues performed a randomized, double-blind trial in patients with a previous history of at least two NMSCs, treating patients with topical tretinoin 0.1 % cream or placebo, and found that the incidence of AKs, BCCs, and SCCs was comparable to the control group [69]. Therefore, the use of topical retinoids as chemopreventive agents is not currently evidence based.

6.3.3 Photodynamic Therapy

Photodynamic therapy (PDT) has been studied as a possible chemopreventive strategy by decreasing the number of actinic keratosis. There are several investigations showing PDT's efficacy in treating AKs; however, reported studies on its use in OTRs are limited [73, 74]. One study in OTRs found a significantly lower incidence of SCCs with cyclic PDT with aminolevulinic acid (ALA) and blue light occurring in 4–8-week intervals [75]. One notable study, by Wulf et al., conducted in 27 renal transplant patients who underwent a single methyl aminolevulinate (MAL)-PDT treatment with red light, showed an increased mean time to onset of new lesions (AKs, SCCs, BCCs, and warts) and an increased number of skin areas remaining free of new lesions [76]. Conversely, another study, which did differentiate NMSCs from keratotic skin lesions, failed to show a reduction in the incidence of SCCs in OTRs undergoing treatment with PDT [77]. Larger studies are needed to confirm the efficacy of PDT as a chemopreventive treatment. Until then, PDT may be considered in areas of field cancerization in OTRs who are unable to tolerate or have contraindications to oral retinoids [44].

6.3.4 Immunosuppressive and Voriconazole Regimens

Modification of immunosuppressive medications is part of the chemopreventive strategy in OTRs with high-risk cutaneous squamous cell carcinomas and those with significant tumor burden [50, 78]. Reducing immunosuppression may decrease overall tumor burden, risk for metastasis, and development of new skin cancers [50]. Dantal and colleagues performed a randomized control trial, which included 231 renal transplant recipients who were randomized (1 year following the date of transplantation) to either receive a reduced regimen or be continued on their immunosuppressive regimen. The patients who were treated with reduced immunosuppressive dosages developed significantly less tumors. However, these patients also experienced more episodes of acute rejection, which were managed and did not influence graft or overall survival [79]. One report examined the effect of greatly reducing immunosuppressants in OTRs with deeply invasive or metastatic SCC. In this account, four of nine patients were managed with reduction or discontinuation of immunosuppression and all four experienced a significantly longer survival period than those maintained on their regular immunosuppressive regimen [80]. Although one of these four patients died, only one of the three surviving patients experienced graft rejection. As reduction of the level of immunosuppression has been shown to decrease the number of SCC and possibly improve prognosis in patients with life-threatening cutaneous carcinomas, efforts should be taken to reduce patient's immunosuppression to the lowest level while still preserving adequate graft function [45, 44, 50]. Conversely, reduction of immunosuppression is not without risk; therefore, these multidisciplinary decisions must be carefully weighed.

Additionally, clinical data has demonstrated that conversion from a calcineurin inhibitor (CNI)-based immunosuppressive regimen to medications such as sirolimus and everolimus can lead to a reduction of SCC [48, 81–86]. These medications are inhibitors of the mammalian target of rapamycin (mTOR) and at the cellular level have exhibited antiproliferative effects [22]. A multicenter trial assessed the effect of continuing kidney transplant patients on a CNI-based regimen verses changing these OTRs to sirolimus. This group demonstrated that transitioning kidney transplant patients (with a history of at least one SCC) to sirolimus had a beneficial, antitumoral effect. The patients that were changed to an mTOR-based regimen experienced a significantly longer survival free of SCCs. Not only did more patients who were receiving calcineurin inhibitors develop new SCCs, but the time to development of these cutaneous carcinomas was also significantly less (7 verses 15 months). While graft function remained stable in the two study groups, it should be noted that there were more serious adverse events in the sirolimus group forcing 23 % of patients to discontinue the medication as a result of these events [87]. Another study conducted by de Fijter and colleagues assessed 53 renal transplant patients developing NMSCs and found that with the conversion of immunosuppression to sirolimus or everolimus, there was resulting remission of NMSCs in 37 patients [83]. Other trials have also displayed the benefits of treating with sirolimus by demonstrating a reduction in new NSMCs or inducing regression of preexisting lesions [84–86].

While studies have confirmed that the conversion from a CNI-based regimen to sirolimus is safe and has a lower incidence of exacerbating hypertension and nephrotoxicity, there is a high rate of potentially serious side effects associated with sirolimus treatment [22, 88, 89]. Adverse effects with mTOR inhibitors include impaired wound healing, myelosuppression, hyperlipidemia, edema, proteinuria, mucosal ulcers, acneiform eruptions, pneumonitis, and thrombotic microangiopathy. The conversion from a CNI-based immunosuppressive regimen to one based on mTOR inhibition should not occur prior to the completion of surgical wound healing and establishment of graft function [90, 44, 22]. Due to impaired wound healing, risk of hepatic artery thrombosis (in liver transplant recipients), and contraindications such as obesity and proteinuria, sirolimus is not usually initiated immediately following transplantation [22, 89, 91]. While the antineoplastic effects of sirolimus are promising, conversion of CNIs to mTOR inhibitors carries potential adverse reactions and includes the risk of compromising graft function.

Additionally, although not a part of the immunosuppressive regimen, voriconazole has been shown to be linked to development of SCCs in transplant recipients [91]. As OTRs are at an increased risk for infections, they are commonly treated with antimicrobial prophylaxis. Voriconazole is a broad-spectrum antifungal commonly used in the transplant population, especially lung transplant patients, which has been associated with several serious side effects. Voriconazole-induced phototoxicity has been well documented, and a recent study conducted by Singer and colleagues demonstrated a dose-dependent increased risk of SCC in lung transplant recipients who had been exposed to voriconazole [92–94]. Therefore, additional consideration should be employed when continuing voriconazole prophylactically in OTRs with high-risk SCCs, and some have suggested the use of posaconazole, as an alternative, in this population [95].

6.3.5 Other Chemopreventive Agents

Other potential chemopreventive agents have been studied, some with promising but often mixed results. These include nonsteroidal anti-inflammatory drugs (NSAIDs), difluoromethylornithine (DFMO), T4 endonuclease V, polyphenols, capecitabine, vitamin D, and other various dietary changes [96–107]. There are a few small studies on organ transplant patients. One study conducted with OTRs found that there were no invasive SCCs discovered in areas treated with topical diclofenac sodium (a cyclooxygenase 2 inhibitor) within a 2-year follow-up period [103]. Additionally, DFMO, which inhibits an enzyme that is induced by ultraviolet irradiation, has been shown to be safe and effective in decreasing AKs in OTRs. Although it was not initially shown to be effective in reducing new NMSCs in this population, a subsequent analysis assessing BCCs and SCCs separately displayed a significant reduction in the development of new BCCs but no difference in SCC development, imparting potential as a chemopreventive [102]. Ten solid OTRs who were treated with low doses of capecitabine experienced a decline in the average incidence rate of SCCs per month (during the first 12 months of treatment) [107]. More studies are needed to confirm the role of these potential agents, and studies specifically in OTRs are lacking.

Other agents still require more research prior to being considered as potential chemopreventive agents. These include perillyl alcohol (POH), peroxisome proliferator-activated receptors (PPARs), genistein, curcumin, silymarin, and lycopene [108]. Theoretically, topicals such as 5-fluorouracil, imiquimod, and ingenol mebutate may decrease the risk of SCCs through their treatment of precancerous AKs [44]. The chemopreventive role of topical imiquimod and ingenol mebutate has not been investigated, but topical 5-fluorouracil is currently being assessed as a preventive agent for NMSC in high-risk populations [109].

Several agents have failed to show benefit as chemopreventive agents for NMSC. These include vitamin E, beta-carotene, selenium, and statins [110–112].

References

1. Brantsch KD, Meisner C, Schönfisch B, Trilling B, Wehner-Caroli J, Röcken M, et al. Analysis of risk factors determining prognosis of cutaneous squamous-cell carcinoma: a prospective study. Lancet Oncol. 2008;9:713–20.

2. Schmults CD, Karia PS, Crter JB, Han J, Qureshi AA. Factors predictive of recurrence and death from cutaneous squamous cell carcinoma. JAMA Dermatol. 2013;149:541–7.
3. Krynitz B, Edgren G, Lindelöf B, Baecklund E, Brattström C, Wilczek H, Smedby KE. Risk of skin cancer and other malignancies in kidney, liver, heart and lung transplant recipients 1970 to 2008—a Swedish population-based study. Int J Cancer. 2013;132:1429–38. doi:10.1002/ijc.27765.
4. London NJ, Farmery SM, et al. Risk of neoplasia in renal transplant patients. Lancet. 1995;346:403–6.
5. Euvrard S, Kanitakis J, Claudy A. Skin cancers after organ transplantation. N Engl J Med. 2003;348:1681–91.
6. Prado R, Francis SO, Mason MN, Wing G, Gamble RG, Dellavalle R. Nonmelanoma skin cancer chemoprevention. Dermatol Surg. 2011;37(11):1566–78.
7. Berg D, Otley CC. Skin cancer in organ transplant recipients: epidemiology, pathogenesis, and management. J Am Acad Dermatol. 2002;47:1–17; quiz 18–20.
8. Zwald FO, Brown M. Skin cancer in solid organ transplant recipients: advances in therapy and management: part I. Epidemiology of skin cancer in solid organ transplant recipients. J Am Acad Dermatol. 2011;65(2):253–61; quiz 262.
9. Cutaneous squamous cell carcinoma and other cutaneous carcinomas. In: Edge SB, Byrd DR, Compton CC, et al., editors. AJCC cancer staging manual. 7th ed. New York: Springer; 2010. p. 301–14.
10. Carcinoma of the eyelid. In: Edge SB, Byrd DR, Compton CC, et al., editors. AJCC cancer staging manual. 7th ed. New York: Springer; 2010. p. 523–6.
11. Jambusaria-Pahlajani A, Kanetsky PA, Karia PS, et al. Evaluation of AJCC tumor staging for cutaneous squamous cell carcinoma and a proposed alternative tumor staging system. JAMA Dermatol. 2013;149(4):402–10.
12. Karia PS, Jambusaria-Pahlajani A, Harrington DP, et al. Evaluation of American Joint Committee on Cancer, International Union Against Cancer, and Brigham and Women's Hospital tumor staging for cutaneous squamous cell carcinoma. J Clin Oncol. 2014;32(4):327–34.
13. Martorell-Calatayud A, Sanmartin Jimenez O, Cruz Mojarrieta J, et al. Cutaneous squamous cell carcinoma: defining the high-risk variant. Actas Dermosifiliogr. 2013;104:367–79.
14. Zwald F. Toward a better definition of high-risk cutaneous squamous cell carcinoma comment on "factors predictive of recurrence and death from cutaneous squamous cell carcinoma". JAMA Dermatol. 2013;149(5):547–8.
15. Huang C, Boyce SM. Surgical margins of excision for basal cell carcinoma and squamous cell carcinoma. Semin Cutan Med Surg. 2004;23:167–73.
16. Clayman GL, Lee JL, Holsinger C, Zhou X, Duvic M, El-Naggar AK, et al. Mortality risk from squamous cell skin cancer. J Clin Oncol. 2005;22:759.
17. Breuninger H, Schaumburg-Lever G, Holzschuh J, Horny HP. Desmoplastic squamous cell carcinoma of skin and vermilion surface. A highly malignant subtype of skin cancer. Cancer. 1997;79:915–9.
18. Farasat S, Yu SS, Neel VA, et al. A new American Joint Committee on Cancer staging system for cutaneous squamous cell carcinoma: creation and rationale for inclusion of tumor (T) characteristics. J Am Acad Dermatol. 2011;64:1051–9.
19. O'Bryan K, Sherman W, Niedt GW, et al. An evolving paradigm for the workup and management of high-risk cutaneous squamous cell carcinoma. J Am Acad Dermatol. 2013;69:595–602.
20. Metchnikoff C, Mully T, Singer JP, Golden JA, Arron ST. The 7th edition AJCC staging system for cutaneous squamous cell carcinoma accurately predicts risk of recurrence for heart and lung transplant recipients. J Am Acad Dermatol. 2012;67(5):829–35. doi:10.1016/j.jaad.2012.01.010. Epub 2012 Jan 29.
21. Veness MJ, Palme CE, Morgan GJ. High-risk cutaneous squamous cell carcinoma of the head and neck: results from 266 treated patients with metastatic lymph node disease. Cancer. 2006;106:2389–96.
22. Martinez JC, Otley CC, Stasko T, Euvrard S, et al. Defining the clinical course of metastatic skin cancer in organ transplant recipients: a multicenter collaborative study. Arch Dermatol. 2003;139:301–6.
23. Nguyen P, Vin-Christian K, Ming ME, Berger T. Aggressive squamous cell carcinomas in persons infected with the human immunodeficiency virus. Arch Dermatol. 2002;138:758–63.
24. National Comprehensive Cancer Network. NCCN clinical practice guidelines in oncology: basal and squamous cell skin cancers. Version 2.2013. http://www.nccn.org/professionals/physician_gls/pdf/nmsc.pdf. Accessed 13 Oct 2013.
25. Rowe DE, Carroll RJ, Day CD. Prognostic factors for local recurrence, metastasis, and survival rates in squamous cell carcinoma of the skin, ear and lip. J Am Acad Dermatol. 1992;26:976–90.
26. Grover R, Douglas RG, Shaw HFS. Carcinoma of the lip in Auckland, New Zealand, 1969–1987. Head Neck. 1989;11:264–8.
27. Dinehart SM, Pollack SV. Metastases from squamous cell carcinoma of the skin and lip: an analysis of twenty-seven cases. J Am Acad Dermatol. 1989;21:241–8.
28. Khanna M, Fortier-Riberdy G, Smoller B, Dinehart S. Reporting tumor thickness for cutaneous squamous cell carcinoma. J Cutan Pathol. 2002;29:321–3.
29. Breuninger H, Black B, Rassner G. Microstaging of squamous cell carcinomas. Am J Clin Pathol. 1990;94:624–7.
30. Cherpelis B, Marcusen C, Lang PG. Prognostic factors for metastasis in squamous cell carcinoma of the skin. Dermatol Surg. 2002;28:268.
31. Leibovitch I, Huilgol SC, Selva D, Hill D, Richards S, Paver R. Cutaneous squamous cell carcinoma treated with Mohs micrographic surgery in Australia II. Perineural invasion. J Am Acad Dermatol. 2005;53:261–6.

32. Goepfert H, Dichtel WJ, Medina JE, Lindberg RD, Luna MD. Perineural invasion in squamous cell skin carcinoma of the head and neck. Am J Surg. 1984;148:542–7.
33. Mendenhall WM, Ferlito A, Takes RP, et al. Cutaneous head and neck basal and squamous cell carcinomas with perineural invasion. Review. Oral Oncol. 2012;48:918–22.
34. Ross AS, Whalllen FM, Elenitsas R, Xu X, Troxel A, Schmults CD. Diameter of involved nerves predicts outcomes in cutaneous squamous cell carcinoma with perineural invasion: an investigator-blinded retrospective cohort study. Dermatol Surg. 2009;35:1859–66.
35. Carter JB, Johnson MM, Chua TL, Karia PS, Schmults CD. Outcomes of primary cutaneous squamous cell carcinoma with perineural invasion: an 11-year cohort study. JAMA Dermatol. 2013;149:35–42.
36. Moore B, Weber RS, Prieto V, El-Naggar A, Holsinger FC, Zhou X, et al. Lymph node metastases from cutaneous squamous cell carcinoma of the head and neck. Laryngoscope. 2006;115:1561.
37. Toll A, Gimeno-Beltrán J, Ferrandiz-Pulido C, Masferrer E, Yébenes M, Jucglà A, Abal L, Martí RM, Sanmartín O, Baró T, Casado B, Gandarillas A, Barranco C, Costa I, Mojal S, García-Patos V, Pujol RM. D2-40 immunohistochemical overexpression in cutaneous squamous cell carcinomas: a marker of metastatic risk. J Am Acad Dermatol. 2012;67(6):1310–8. doi:10.1016/j.jaad.2012.03.007. Epub 2012 Apr 20.
38. Chang S, Low I, Ng D, Brasch H, Sullivan M, Davis P, et al. Epidermal growth factor receptor: a novel biomarker for aggressive head and neck cutaneous squamous cell carcinoma. Hum Pathol. 2008;39:34.
39. American Cancer Society. Cancer Facts & Figures 2013. http://www.cancer.org/acs/groups/content/@epidemiologysurveilance/documents/document/acspc-036845.pdf. Accessed 21 Oct 2013.
40. Armstrong BK, Kricker A. The epidemiology of UV induced skin cancer. J Photochem Photobiol B. 2001;63:8–18.
41. Wright TI, Spencer JM, Flowers FP. Chemoprevention of nonmelanoma skin cancer. J Am Acad Dermatol. 2006;54:933–46; quiz 47–50.
42. Sporn MB. Approaches to prevention of epithelial cancer during the preneoplastic period. Cancer Res. 1976;36(7 PT 2):2699–702.
43. Bowden GT. Prevention of non-melanoma skin cancer by targeting ultraviolet-B-light signaling. Nat Rev Cancer. 2004;4(1):23–35.
44. Soltani-Arabshahi R, Tristani-Firouz P. Chemoprevention of nonmelanoma skin cancer. Facial Plast Surg. 2013;29(05):373–83.
45. Otley CC, Stasko T, Tope WD, Lebwohl M. Chemoprevention of nonmelanoma skin cancer with systemic retinoids: practical dosing and management of adverse effects. Dermatol Surg. 2006;32(4):562–8.
46. Jensen AO, Svaerke C, Farkas D, Pedersen L, Kragballe K, Sørensen HT. Skin cancer risk among solid organ recipients: a nationwide cohort study in Denmark. Acta Derm Venereol. 2010;90(5):474–9.
47. Collett D, Mumford L, Banner NR, Neuberger J, Watson C. Comparison of the incidence of malignancy in recipients of different types of organ: a UK Registry audit. Am J Transplant. 2010;10(8):1889–96.
48. Euvrard S, Kanitakis J, Decullier E, et al. Subsequent skin cancers in kidney and heart transplant recipients after the first squamous cell carcinoma. Transplantation. 2006;81(8):1093–100.
49. Mehrany K, Weenig RH, Lee KK, Pittelkow MR, Otley CC. Increased metastasis and mortality from cutaneous squamous cell carcinoma in patients with chronic lymphocytic leukemia. J Am Acad Dermatol. 2005;53(6):1067–71.
50. Otley CC, Cherikh WS, Salasche SJ, McBride MA, Christenson LJ, Kauffman HM. Skin cancer in organ transplant recipients: effect of pretransplant end-organ disease. J Am Acad Dermatol. 2005;53(5):783–90.
51. Patton TJ, Zirwas MJ, Wolverton SE. Systemic retinoids. 2nd ed. Philadelphia: Elsevier; 2007.
52. Altucci L, et al. The promise of retinoids to fight against cancer. Nat Rev Cancer. 2001;1:181–93.
53. Lens M, Medenica L. Systemic retinoids in chemoprevention of non-melanoma skin cancer. Expert Opin Pharmacother. 2008;9:1363–74.
54. Levine N. Role of retinoids in skin cancer treatment and prevention. J Am Acad Dermatol. 1998;39:S62–6.
55. Hong WK, Sporn MB. Recent advances in chemoprevention of cancer. Science. 1997;278(5340):1073–7.
56. Mrass P, Rendl M, Mildner M, Gruber F, et al. Retinoic acid increases the expression of p53 and proapoptotic caspases and sensitizes keratinocytes to apoptosis: a possible explanation for tumor preventive action of retinoids. Cancer Res. 2004;64:6542–8.
57. Clarke N, Germain P, Altucci L, Gronemeyer H. Retinoids: potential in cancer prevention and therapy. Expert Rev Mol Med. 2004;6(25):1–23.
58. Moon TE, Levine N, Cartmel B, et al. Southwest Skin Cancer Prevention Study Group. Effect of retinol in preventing squamous cell skin cancer in moderate-risk subjects: a randomized, double-blind, controlled trial. Cancer Epidemiol Biomarkers Prev. 1997;6(11):949–56.
59. Kraemer KH, DiGiovanna JJ, Moshell AN, Tarone RE, Peck GL. Prevention of skin cancer in xeroderma pigmentosum with the use of oral isotretinoin. N Engl J Med. 1988;318(25):1633–7.
60. Bavinck JN, Tieben LM, Van der Woude FJ, et al. Prevention of skin cancer and reduction of keratotic skin lesions during acitretin therapy in renal transplant recipients: a double-blind, placebo-controlled study. J Clin Oncol. 1995;13(8):1933–8.
61. Tangrea JA, Edwards BK, Taylor PR, et al. Isotretinoin-Basal Cell Carcinoma Study Group. Long-term therapy with low-dose isotretinoin for prevention of basal cell carcinoma: a multicenter clinical trial. J Natl Cancer Inst. 1992;84(5):328–32.
62. McKenna DB, Murphy GM. Skin cancer chemoprophylaxis in renal transplant recipients: 5 years of

experience using low-dose acitretin. Br J Dermatol. 1999;140(4):656–60.
63. Levine N, Moon TE, Cartmel B, et al. Southwest Skin Cancer Prevention Study Group. Trial of retinol and isotretinoin in skin cancer prevention: a randomized, double-blind, controlled trial. Cancer Epidemiol Biomarkers Prev. 1997;6(11):957–61.
64. Nijsten TE, Stern RS. Oral retinoid use reduces cutaneous squamous cell carcinoma risk in patients with psoriasis treated with psoralen-UVA: a nested cohort study. J Am Acad Dermatol. 2003;49(4):644–50.
65. George R, Weightman W, Russ GR, Bannister KM, Mathew TH. Acitretin for chemoprevention of nonmelanoma skin cancers in renal transplant recipients. Australas J Dermatol. 2002;43(4):269–73.
66. de Sévaux RG, Smit JV, de Jong EM, van de Kerkhof PC, Hoitsma AJ. Acitretin treatment of premalignant and malignant skin disorders in renal transplant recipients: clinical effects of a randomized trial comparing two doses of acitretin. J Am Acad Dermatol. 2003;49(3):407–12.
67. Harwood CA, Leedham-Green M, Leigh IM, Proby CM. Low-dose retinoids in the prevention of cutaneous squamous cell carcinomas in organ transplant recipients: a 16-year retrospective study. Arch Dermatol. 2005;141(4):456–64.
68. Gibson GE, O'Grady A, Kay EW, Murphy GM. Low-dose retinoid therapy for chemoprophylaxis of skin cancer in renal transplant recipients. J Eur Acad Dermatol Venereol. 1998;10(1):42–7.
69. Weinstock MA, Bingham SF, Digiovanna JJ, et al. Veterans Affairs Topical Tretinoin Chemoprevention Trial Group. Tretinoin and the prevention of keratinocyte carcinoma (Basal and squamous cell carcinoma of the skin): a veterans affairs randomized chemoprevention trial. J Invest Dermatol. 2012;132(6):1583–90.
70. Peris K, Fargnoli MC, Chimenti S. Preliminary observations on the use of topical tazarotene to treat basal-cell carcinoma. N Engl J Med. 1999;341(23):1767–8.
71. Bardazzi F, Bianchi F, Parente G, Guareschi E, Landi C. A pilot study on the use of topical tazarotene to treat squamous cell carcinoma in situ. J Am Acad Dermatol. 2005;52(6):1102–4.
72. Smit JV, Cox S, Blokx WA, van de Kerhof PC, de Jongh GJ, de Jong EM. Actinic keratoses in renal transplant recipients do not improve with calcipotriol cream and all-trans retinoic acid cream as monotherapies or in combination during a 6-week treatment period. Br J Dermatol. 2002;147(4):816–8.
73. Varma S, Wilson H, Kurwa HA, et al. Bowen's disease, solar keratoses and superficial basal cell carcinomas treated by photodynamic therapy using a large-field incoherent light source. Br J Dermatol. 2001;144(3):567–74.
74. Markham T, Collins P. Topical 5-aminolaevulinic acid photodynamic therapy for extensive scalp actinic keratoses. Br J Dermatol. 2001;145:502–4.
75. Willey A, Mehta S, Lee PK. Reduction in the incidence of squamous cell carcinoma in solid organ transplant recipients treated with cyclic photodynamic therapy. Dermatol Surg. 2010;36(5):652–8.
76. Wulf HC, Pavel S, Stender I, Bakker-Wensveen CA. Topical photodynamic therapy for prevention of new skin lesions in renal transplant recipients. Acta Derm Venereol. 2006;86(1):25–8.
77. de Graaf YG, Kennedy C, Wolterbeek R, Collen AF, Willemze R, Bouwes Bavinck JN. Photodynamic therapy does not prevent cutaneous squamous-cell carcinoma in organ-transplant recipients: results of a randomized-controlled trial. J Invest Dermatol. 2006;126(3):569–74.
78. Neuberg M. Transplant-associated skin cancer: role of reducing immunosuppression. J Natl Compr Canc Netw. 2007;5(5):541–9.
79. Dantal J, Hourmant M, Cantarovich D, et al. Effect of long-term immunosuppression in kidney-graft recipients on cancer incidence: randomized comparison of two cyclosporin regimens. Lancet. 1998;351:623–8.
80. Moloney FJ, Kelly PO, Kay EW, et al. Maintenance versus reduction of immunosuppression in renal transplant recipients with aggressive squamous cell carcinoma. Dermatol Surg. 2004;30:674–8.
81. Kauffman HM, Cherikh WS, Cheng Y, Hanto DW, Kahan BD. Maintenance immunosuppression with target-of-rapamycin inhibitors is associated with a reduced incidence of de novo malignancies. Transplantation. 2005;80(7):883–9.
82. Yakupoglu YK, Buell JF, Woodle S, Kahan BD. Individualization of immunosuppressive therapy. III. Sirolimus associated with a reduced incidence of malignancy. Transplant Proc. 2006;38(2):358–61.
83. de Fijter JW. Use of proliferation signal inhibitors in non-melanoma skin cancer following renal transplantation. Nephrol Dial Transplant. 2007;22 Suppl 01:i23–6.
84. Rival-Tringali AL, Euvrard S, Decullier E, Claudy A, et al. Conversion from calcineurin inhibitors to sirolimus reduces vascularization and thickness of post-transplant cutaneous squamous cell carcinomas. Anticancer Res. 2009;29:1927–32.
85. Salgo R, Gossmann J, Schofer H, Kachel HG, et al. Switch to sirolimus-based immunosuppression in long-term renal transplant recipients: reduced rate of (pre-) malignancies and nonmelanoma skin cancer in a prospective, randomized, assessor-blinded, controlled clinical trial. Am J Transplant. 2010;10:1385–93.
86. Tessmer CS, Magalhães LV, Keitel E, Valar C, et al. Conversion to sirolimus in renal transplant recipients with skin cancer. Transplantation. 2006;82:1792–3.
87. Euvrard S, Morelon E, Rostaing L, et al. Sirolimus and secondary skin-cancer prevention in kidney transplantation. N Engl J Med. 2012;367(4):329–39.
88. Diekmann F, Campistol JM. Conversion from calcineurin inhibitors to sirolimus in chronic allograft nephropathy: benefits and risks. Nephrol Dial Transplant. 2006;21:562–8.
89. Peddi VR, Jensik S, Pescovitx M, Pirsch J, et al. An open-label, pilot study evaluating the safety and efficacy of converting from calcineurin inhibitors to sirolimus in established renal allograft recipients with moderate renal insufficiency. Clin Transplant. 2005;19:130–6.

90. Augustine JJ, Bodziak KA, Hricik DE. Use of sirolimus in solid organ transplantation. Drugs. 2007;67(3):369–91.
91. Massoud O, Wiesner RH. The use of sirolimus should be restricted in liver transplantation. J Hepatol. 2012;56(1):288–90.
92. Singer JP, Boker A, Metchnikoff C, et al. High cumulative dose exposure to voriconazole is associated with cutaneous squamous cell carcinoma in lung transplant recipients. J Heart Lung Transplant. 2012;31:694–9.
93. Cowen EW, Nguyen JC, Miller DD, et al. Chronic phototoxicity and aggressive squamous cell carcinoma of the skin in children and adults during treatment with voriconazole. J Am Acad Dermatol. 2010;62:31–7.
94. McCarthy KL, Playford EG, Looke DF, Whitby M. Severe photosensitivity causing multifocal squamous cell carcinomas secondary to prolonged voriconazole therapy. Clin Infect Dis. 2007;44:e55–6.
95. Vanacker A, Fabre G, Van Dorpe J, Peetermans WE, Maes B. Aggressive cutaneous squamous cell carcinoma associated with prolonged voriconazole therapy in a renal transplant patient. Am J Transplant. 2008;8:877–80.
96. An KP, Athar M, Tang X, et al. Cyclooxygenase-2 expression in murine and human nonmelanoma skin cancers: implications for therapeutic approaches. Photochem Photobiol. 2002;76(1):73–80.
97. Higashi Y, Kanckura T, Kanzaki T. Enhanced expression of cyclooxygenase (COX)-2 in human skin epidermal cancer cells: evidence for growth suppression by inhibiting COX-2 expression. Int J Cancer. 2000;86(5):667–71.
98. Asgari MM, Chren MM, Warton EM, Friedman GD, et al. Association between nonsteroidal anti-inflammatory drug use and cutaneous squamous cell carcinoma. Arch Dermatol. 2010;146:388–95.
99. Butler GJ, Neale R, Green AC, Pandeya N, Whiteman DC. Nonsteroidal anti-inflammatory drugs and the risk of actinic keratoses and squamous cell cancers of the skin. J Am Acad Dermatol. 2005;53(6):966–72.
100. Elmets CA, Viner JL, Pentland AP, Cantrell W, et al. Chemoprevention of nonmelanoma skin cancer with celecoxib: a randomized, double-blind, placebo-controlled trial. J Natl Cancer Inst. 2010;102:1835–44.
101. Torti DC, Christensen BC, Storm CA, et al. Analgesic and nonsteroidal anti-inflammatory use in relation to nonmelanoma skin cancer: a population-based case–control study. J Am Acad Dermatol. 2011;65(2):304–12.
102. Bailey HH, Kim K, Verma AK, et al. A randomized, double-blind, placebo-controlled phase 3 skin cancer prevention study of alpha-difluoromethylornithine in subjects with previous history of skin cancer. Cancer Prev Res (Phila). 2010;3(1):35–47.
103. Yarosh D, Klein J, O'Connor A, Hawk J, Rafal E, Wolf P. Xeroderma Pigmentosum Study Group. Effect of topically applied T4 endonuclease V in liposomes on skin cancer in xeroderma pigmentosum: a randomized study. Lancet. 2001;357(9260):926–9.
104. Ulrich C, Johannsen A, Röwert-Huber J, Ulrich M, Sterry W, Stockfleth E. Results of a randomized, placebo-controlled safety and efficacy study of topical diclofenac 3 % gel in organ transplant patients with multiple actinic keratoses. Eur J Dermatol. 2010;20(4):482–8.
105. Gandini S, Raimondi S, Gnagnarella P, Doré JF, Maisonneuve P, Testori A. Vitamin D and skin cancer: a meta-analysis. Eur J Cancer. 2009;45(4):634–41.
106. Song F, Qureshi AA, Han J. Increased caffeine intake is associated with reduced risk of basal cell carcinoma of the skin. Cancer Res. 2012;72(13):3282–9.
107. Endrizzi B, Ahmad RL, Ray T, Dudek A, Lee P. Capecitabine to reduce nonmelanoma skin carcinoma burden in solid organ transplant recipients. Dermatol Surg. 2013;39(4):634–45.
108. Jee SH, et al. Curcumin induces a p53-dependent apoptosis in human basal cell carcinoma cells. J Invest Dermatol. 1998;111:656–61.
109. Weiss J, Menter A, Hevia O, Ling M, et al. Effective treatment of actinic keratosis with 0.5 % fluorouracil cream for 1, 2, or 4 weeks. Cutis. 2002;70:22–9.
110. Frieling UM, et al. A randomized, 12-year primary-prevention trial of beta carotene supplementation for nonmelanoma skin cancer in the physician's health study. Arch Dermatol. 2000;136:179–84.
111. Greenberg ER, et al. A clinical trial of beta-carotene to prevent basal cell and squamous-cell cancers of the skin. N Engl J Med. 1990;323:789–95.
112. Asgari MM, et al. Statin use and risk of basal cell carcinoma. JAAD. 2009;61:66–72.

7 Advances in Management of "High-Risk Squamous Cell Carcinoma" in Organ Transplant Recipients

Mary L. Stevenson and John A. Carucci

Contents

M.L. Stevenson, MD (✉)
The Ronald O. Perelman Department of Dermatology, NYU Langone Medical Center, New York, NY, USA
e-mail: mary.stevenson@nyumc.org

J.A. Carucci, MD
The Ronald O. Perelman Department of Dermatology, NYU Dermatological Surgical Associates, New York, NY, USA
e-mail: john.carucci@nyumc.org

Abbreviations

5-FU	5-Fuorouracil
BCC	Basal cell carcinoma
IL-2	Interleukin-2
MMF	Mycophenolate mofetil
NMSC	Nonmelanoma skin cancer
OTR	Organ transplant recipient
SCC	Squamous cell carcinoma
SLNB	Sentinel lymph node biopsy

7.1 Introduction

There are an estimated 130,000 living organ transplant recipients (OTRs) in the United States [1]. Kidney transplants are the most common, followed by the liver, heart, lung, and subsequently multiorgan transplants including the pancreas and intestine. Since the first successful kidney transplant in 1954, major advances in the field of transplantation have led to increased long-term survival among OTRs. Improved immunosuppressive therapy, increased treatment of infectious diseases, and better human leukocyte antigen matching has led to decreased rejection and longer patient survival [2–4]. These patients are at an increased risk for the development of skin cancer and require careful consideration and management by dermatologists.

F. Zwald, M.D. Brown (eds.), *Advances in Transplant Dermatology: Clinical and Practical Implications*, DOI 10.1007/978-3-319-12445-2_7, © Springer International Publishing Switzerland 2015

7.2 Epidemiology

OTRs are at an increased risk for cutaneous malignancy, particularly squamous cell carcinoma (SCC) and basal cell carcinoma (BCC) which account for 95 % of all skin cancers in OTRs [2, 5, 6]. They are also at increased risk for melanoma, Merkel cell carcinoma, and Kaposi's sarcoma [2, 5–8]. SCC causes significant morbidity and mortality in this patient population and is also associated with financial burden and an increased cost of care in OTRs (Fig. 7.1) [9]. In contrast to the general population where BCCs predominate, OTRs have a comparatively increased rate of SCCs [10]. Additionally, the majority of these malignancies occur on sun-exposed sites [10, 11]. In an Australian study of heart transplant recipients, the ratio of SCC to BCC was found to be 3:1 [12]. Skin cancer accounted for 27 % of 41 deaths after the fourth year of transplantation in this study and included six deaths from SCC, four deaths from melanoma, and one death from Merkel cell carcinoma in 400 patients. Additionally fair skin, increased age, HLA-DR homozygosity, and length of time after transplantation were all associated with the development of cutaneous malignancy [12]. This ratio is similar to that found in other studies though the ratio has been quoted to be anywhere from 1.5 to 8.6:1 for SCC to BCCs [5, 13, 14]. Male sex, prior history of skin cancer, and type of transplantation—with heart transplant patients having more malignancies than kidney transplant patients—have also been associated with an increased risk of cutaneous malignancy [11, 15]. A Norwegian study of kidney and heart transplant patients found a 65 % increase in the risk of SCC as compared to the general population and that the risk was associated with the degree of immunosuppression [16, 17].

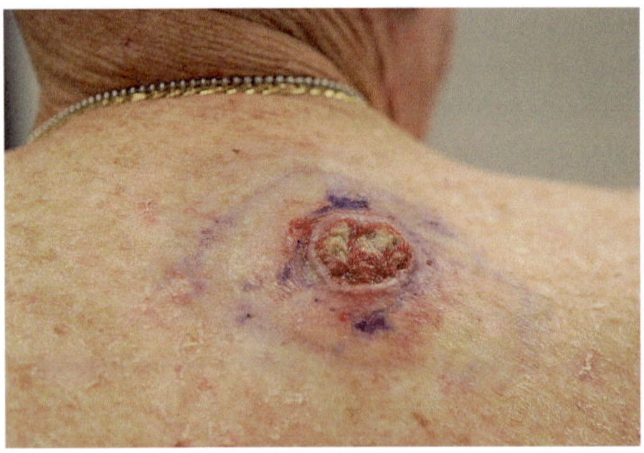

Fig. 7.1 High-risk primary SCC in an organ transplant patient

Moreover, immunosuppression after solid-organ transplantation was originally recognized in the dermatology literature as a risk factor for more aggressive SCC by Rowe in 1992 [18]. Others have confirmed that SCC in OTRs has an increased rate of local recurrence, metastasis, and morbidity [2, 12, 13]. The rate of metastasis of SCC in this population is 7–8 % as compared to 0.5–5 % in the general population [10, 18, 19]. Furthermore, metastasis in the setting of immunosuppression has been associated with a poor prognosis [20]. In-transit metastasis with SCC has also been described more commonly in OTRs and represents a unique, more aggressive presentation of SCC associated with a poor prognosis [21].

7.3 Immunosuppressive Agents

Lifelong immunosuppression prevents graft rejection, and improved regimens have opened the door to increased survival times in the field of organ transplantation. Most immunosuppressive agents, however, have also been associated with an increased risk of malignancy, notably skin cancers. Controversy exists as to which particular agents contribute most to the development of cutaneous malignancy, and there has been some suggestion that older agents including antiproliferative agents such as azathioprine and calcineurin inhibitors (e.g., cyclosporine) may contribute to the development of skin cancers more so than newer agents such as the mTOR inhibitor sirolimus [14, 22]. Little controversy, however, exists that the degree and duration of immunosuppression correlate with the development of aggressive SCC [2, 14]. Induction therapy with a lymphocyte-depleting agent or an interluekin-2 receptor antagonist is given just before, at the time of, or just following organ transplantation to prevent acute rejection [10]. This course is followed by maintenance immunosuppression, which is given in higher doses for the first 3 months posttransplantation when the risk of rejection is highest.

The earliest antirejection protocols from the 1970s traditionally included corticosteroids, azathioprine, and cyclosporine [2]. Azathioprine is a purine analog which acts as a prodrug for mercaptopurine and inhibits the proliferation of T and B cells [23]. Treatment with azathioprine, a potent photosensitizer, increases the skin's susceptibility to damage from UVA radiation [10, 24]. Cyclosporine binds cyclophilin and inhibits calcineurin, preventing activation of interleukin-2 (IL-2) and inhibiting T cell formation [25]. Corticosteroids predominantly inhibit T cell proliferation [26]. Azathioprine, cyclosporine, and prednisolone have all been associated with an increased risk of cutaneous carcinogenesis with the proposed mechanism of decreased immune surveillance as well as possible direct carcinogenesis [2, 27–30]. Induction chemotherapy with OKT3, antithymocyte globulin, or monoclonal anti-IL2 receptor antibodies has also been associated with an increased risk of nonmelanoma skin cancers (NMSCs) [10, 31, 32].

Jensen et al. showed that kidney transplant recipients had a 4.2-fold increased risk of developing SCC while on triple immunosuppression (cyclosporine, azathioprine, and prednisolone) in comparison to those receiving only azathioprine and prednisolone [16, 17]. While Dantal et al. showed that 26 as compared to 17 patients in normal- and low-dose cyclosporine groups, respectively, developed at least one skin cancer correlating the degree of immunosuppression with the risk of malignancy [33]. Another large study in the United Kingdom found increased rates of cutaneous malignancies in renal transplant patients with poor renal function, requiring increased immunosuppression as compared to those receiving organs from a living donor who usually require lower regimens [15]. However, literature has suggested that cyclosporine, rather than diminishing the immune system's response to carcinogenic cells, may in fact lead to non-immune-mediated mechanism of oncogenic development [34]. Hojo et al. found that cyclosporine may promote cancer development and progression through the induction of transforming growth factor-β [28].

Newer immunosuppressive regimens including agents such as mycophenolate mofetil, tacrolimus, and sirolimus have aimed at reducing the morbidity associated with long-term immunosuppression. Mycophenolate mofetil (MMF) inhibits de novo purine synthesis hindering T and B cell proliferation [35], while tacrolimus, a calcineurin inhibitor, also binds the FK-binding protein preventing the activation of IL-2 and therefore the proliferation of B and T cells [3]. Studies have shown a lower incidence of skin cancers in OTRs treated with tacrolimus in comparison to those treated with cyclosporine [36]. In animal studies of UVB-exposed mice, those treated with cyclosporine or tacrolimus developed larger tumors than vehicle-treated mice, while the addition of MMF to cyclosporine (but not tacrolimus) significantly reduced tumor size [37]. Other studies in mice however have shown that tacrolimus may have antiproliferative effects [38]. Currently, maintenance therapy with the calcineurin inhibitor tacrolimus over cyclosporine in combination with mycophenolate mofetil instead of azathioprine is recommended [10].

Sirolimus and everolimus are mTOR inhibitors that also bind to the FK-binding protein and may prevent angiogenesis resulting in decreased tumor size and production [3, 10, 11]. They are non-nephrotoxic and therefore are utilized in patients with cyclosporine and tacrolimus induced nephrotoxicity [10]. Studies have demonstrated a decreased risk of de novo malignancies, especially skin cancers, in transplant patients treated with sirolimus. Kauffman et al. showed that the incidence of de novo posttransplant malignancy with sirolimus or everolimus (another mTOR inhibitor) alone or of these agents in addition to cyclosporine or tacrolimus was 0.6 % versus an incidence of 1.81 % in patients treated with cyclosporine or tacrolimus [39]. In another study, patients on cyclosporine, steroids, and sirolimus who had their cyclosporine withdrawn 3 months posttransplant and their sirolimus troughs doubled while continuing on dual therapy with steroids showed reduced rates of both SCCs and BCCs [40]. Mathew et al. reported on the results from five trials involving sirolimus in posttransplant patients and found that 2 years after transplant those receiving sirolimus with cyclosporine had a lower incidence of skin cancer, while those receiving sirolimus as base therapy had no malignancies compared to 5 % in those being treated with cyclosporine, and that those who were trough level controlled on sirolimus with cessation of cyclosporine had a lower incidence of malignancy than those who remained on both agents [41]. Current recommendation is that sirolimus and everolimus should not be initiated until after graft function has been established [10].

Finally, induction chemotherapy with OKT3, antithymocyte globulin, or monoclonal anti-IL2 receptor antibodies has also been associated with an increase risk of nonmelanoma skin cancers (NMSCs) [10, 31, 32].

7.4 Management

7.4.1 Standard Modalities

The gold standard of treatment in OTRs with SCC is surgical excision. It is also important to remember that SCC in OTRs on immunosuppression is considered a high-risk lesion correlated with increased incidence of local recurrence and metastasis [18]. Therefore, establishing which lesions may be at highest risk for metastasis or recurrence and prioritizing treatment of these lesions are important. In general, high-risk SCCs are characterized by large lesion size, rapid growth, aggressive pattern on histology, recurrence (such as those occurring in a scar), and location on the scalp, lip, or ear [2, 14, 18].

Mohs migrographic surgery has been shown to be associated with a lower frequency of local recurrence in the treatment of SCCs in OTRs and is considered standard of care for all high-risk SCCs, while Mohs or surgical excision may be used for low-risk tumors [18, 42]. Subclinical extension of tumor infiltrates has been shown in SCCs in OTRs, further strengthening the utility of Mohs surgery in this patient population (Fig. 7.2a, b) [43]. In addition, a review of OTRs presenting to a single center for Mohs micrographic surgery showed that OTRs have significantly more cutaneous malignancies referred for Mohs surgery with a reversal of the ratio of BCC to SCC as seen in the general population [44]. This study also showed that OTRs generally have smaller tumors than the general population reflecting a likely lower threshold for screening and referring these patients [44]. Standard excision with postoperative margin assessment may also be used with 6–10 mm margins rather than standard 4 mm margin in high-risk lesions when Mohs surgery is not available, the lesion is larger than what is permissible for removal under local anesthesia, or tissue conservation is not a priority [45, 46].

Additional modalities such as radiation therapy should only be considered in high-risk

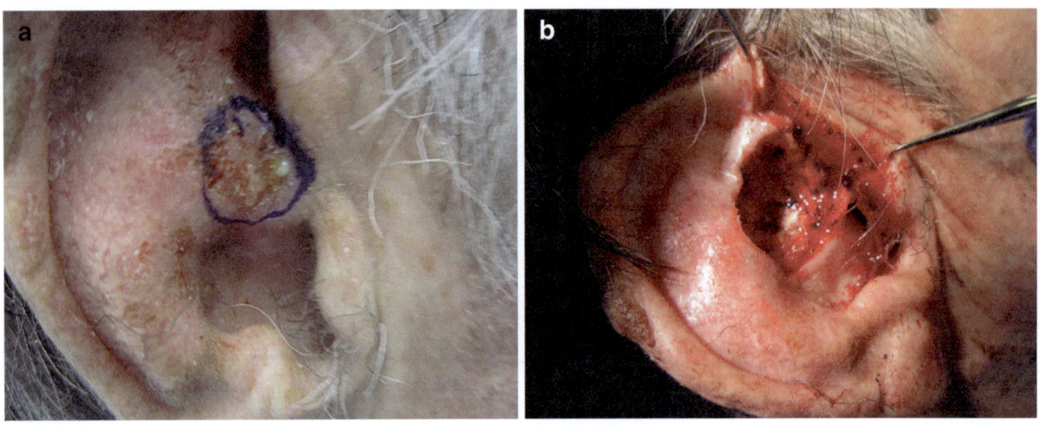

Fig. 7.2 (**a**) High-risk SCC lesion prior to surgical treatment. (**b**) High-risk SCC lesion with deep extension during Mohs excision

lesions if the tumor is inoperable the or patient is unable to undergo surgical excision [46]. However, radiation as an adjunctive treatment may be useful in cases involving perineural invasion [14, 46, 47].

Topical therapies with imiquimod or 5-fluorouracil may be used for in situ SCC lesions or malignant precursors such as actinic keratoses [14, 46]. Electrodessication and curettage may be used for SCC but should not be used for high-risk SCC as it may be associated with potentially higher rate of recurrence [18, 46, 48].

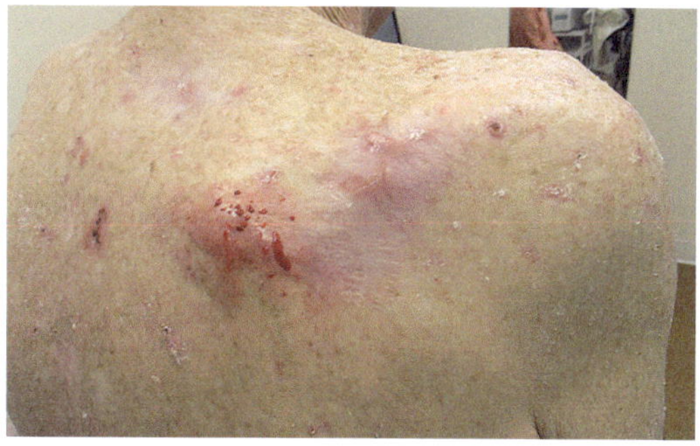

Fig. 7.3 In-transit metastatic SCC to the surrounding skin in a patient with a high-risk primary SCC

7.4.1.1 In-Transit Metastasis

In-transit metastasis is a unique presentation of SCC, most commonly seen in OTRs and associated with a poor prognosis in this population. Representing metastases to the surrounding skin via lymphatic spread, in-transit metastases are a therapeutic challenge in this patient population and must be considered carefully (Fig. 7.3). In one of the first reports on the characteristics of in-transit metastases in cutaneous SCC, a series of 21 patients with in-transit metastasis, (15 of which were OTRs) was reviewed finding that lesions were most often subcutaneous or dermal exophytic papules located in proximity (mean distance of 2.5 cm) to the primary lesion with multiple lesions also being common [21]. In-transit metastases in OTRs in this series was associated with a poor prognosis with only 33 % of patient achieving disease control at 24 months with traditional treatment modalities of Mohs surgical excision, standard excision, excision and radiation, radiation alone, or in a limited number of cases systemic or intralesional chemotherapy [21]. The mean time to development of in-transit metastasis in this review was 10 weeks, while the majority of regional metastasis occurs typically within one and a half years of the primary tumor being diagnosed [21, 49]. Additionally one-third of these patients were alive with either nodal disease or distant metastases at 24 months in comparison to 80 % of the non-transplant patients achieving control with 0 % disease-related mortality at 24 months [21]. As such, in-transit metastases should be handled with a multidisciplinary approach, with surgical excision in addition to consideration for adjuvant radiation therapy or sentinel node biopsy being made on a case-by-case basis [2, 14, 21]. In the experience of these authors, in-transit metastases are routinely removed with surgical excision of the new lesion and adjacent scar from the primary excision, and patients should subsequently be treated with radiation therapy (Table 7.1).

7.4.1.2 "Field Cancerization"

The idea of "field cancerization" in OTRs has been used to describe the extensive areas of actinic damage found in this patient population that are often filled with multiple primary lesions and premalignant precursors or subclinical lesions (Fig. 7.4) [11]. The International Transplant Skin Cancer Collaboration guidelines for the treatment of SCC in OTRs recommend tangential excision followed by cautery for the treatment of in situ SCC for patients with multiple primaries and extensive field disease [46].

Topical therapies and other destructive modalities, such as imiquimod, 5 % fluorouracil (5-FU), and photodynamic therapy, may also be used in concert with excision for patients with extensive areas of malignant and premalignant damage [14, 22]. Imiquimod, approved by the Food and Drug Administration for the treatment of genital warts, actinic keratoses, and superficial basal cell carcinomas, is a nonspecific immunomodulator that has been shown to be safe for use in OTRs on systemic immunosuppression [42, 50]. Topical 5-FU works via inhibition of thymidylate synthase which inhibits

Table 7.1 Management of high-risk SCC in OTRs

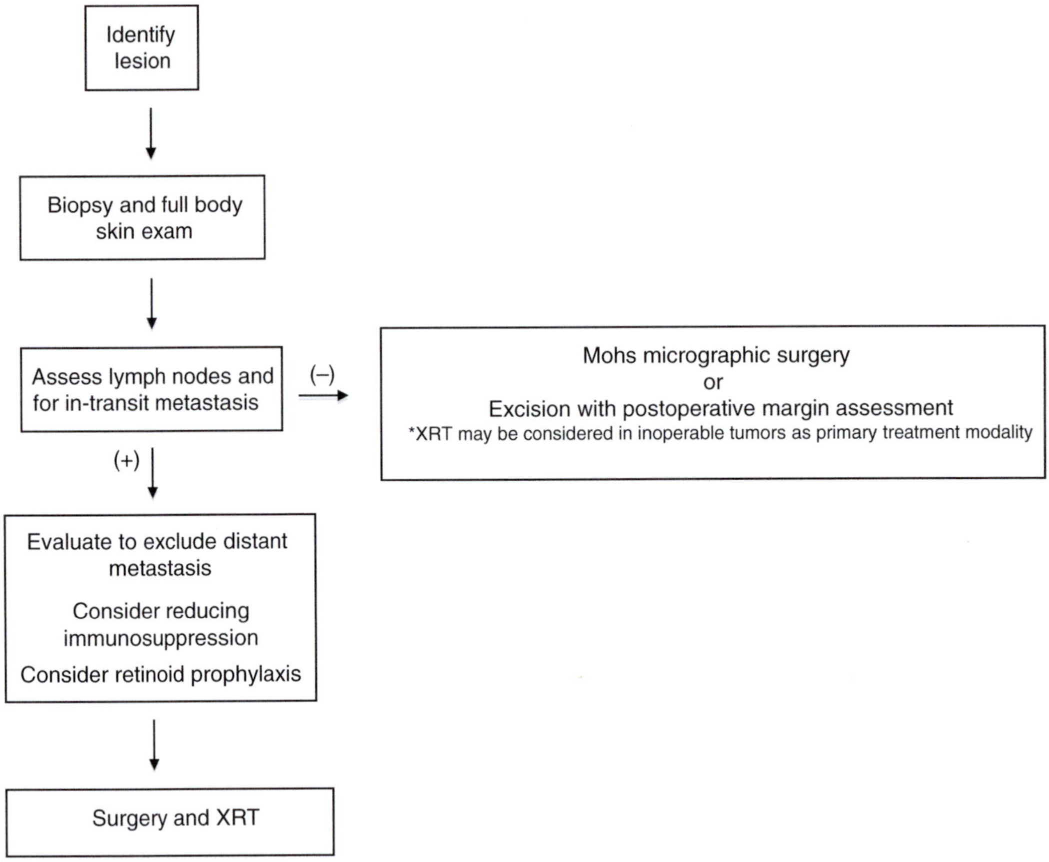

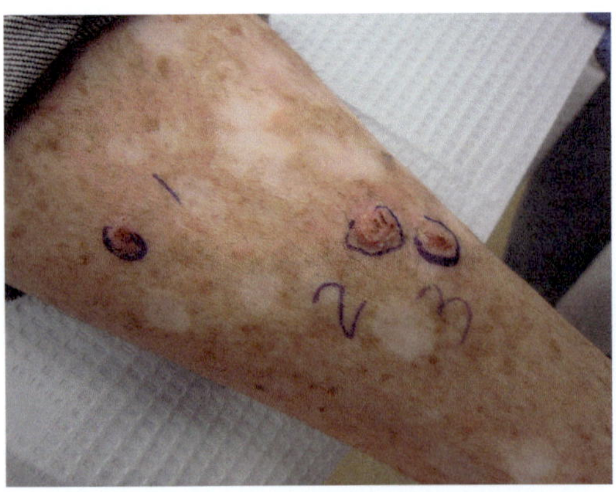

Fig. 7.4 Extensive field cancerization with background actinic damage and multiple primary lesions

DNA synthesis and is the most widely used topical agent for extensive epidermal dysplasia though few studies have evaluated its efficacy in the OTR population [51]. In one study that examined the combination of imiquimod with 5-FU for biopsy-proven in situ SCCs in OTRs, clearing was reported and it was suggested that imiquimod may improve the efficacy of 5-FU [52]. Interestingly, in a small trial comparing 5-FU to photodynamic therapy—which involves the application of photosensitizer such as methylaminolaevulinate or aminolevulinic acid followed by phototherapy—photodynamic therapy was more efficacious and preferred by OTRs for the treatment of epidermal dysplasia extensive field damage [24].

7.4.2 Retinoid Therapy

Retinoids have also been reported as effective chemoprophylaxis for the prevention of skin cancers in OTRs. In this regard, acitretin is preferred over isotretinoin due to a more favorable side effect profile [14]. In a series of five heart transplant recipients with multiple NMSCs, the addition of low-dose acitretin (10 or 25 mg/day) in all five patients resulted in a reduction in the development of premalignant actinic keratoses [53]. In another study of low-dose acitretin (0.3 mg/kg/daily), 12 of 16 patients showed significant reduction in new carcinomas for up to 4 years of treatment of patients with five or more SCCs prior to acitretin therapy benefiting most [54]. In a larger series of 44 renal transplant patients, the addition of 30 mg/day of acitretin decreased the incidence of SCC as well as reducing the occurrence of actinic keratoses, with the effect being most pronounced in those patients with a history of NMSCs [55]. Systemic retinoid therapy, therefore, should be considered in any patient who develops 5–10 SCCs per year, with a lower threshold considered in OTRs with extensive field damage or a history of more aggressive SCCs [42].

7.4.2.1 Sirolimus

Recent investigations into the use of the mTOR inhibitor sirolimus have suggested it may reduce cutaneous SCCs in OTRs. Hoogendijk-van den Akker et al. examined conversion to sirolimus in renal transplant patients with a history of at least one biopsy-proven SCC and found a nonsignificant 24 % reduction in risk of SCCS, with a significant 50 % reduction in the first year [56]. Similar studies by Campbell et al. and Euvrard et al. showed that conversion from calcineurin inhibitors to sirolimus decreased the incidence of new SCCs [57, 58]. Importantly, the studies by Hoogendijk-van den Akker et al. and Euvrard et al. found that the greatest reduction in the development of SCCs occurred early on in the first 1–2 years following conversion. Additionally they found a nonsignificant reduction in the number of subsequent SCCs in patients who had numerous SCCs prior to conversion suggesting that conversion to sirolimus should potentially be considered earlier than the current International Transplant Skin Cancer Collaborative guidelines which recommend conversion only following the development of numerous SCCs, a high-risk SCC, or an SCC with in-transit or metastatic disease [56, 58, 59].

7.4.2.2 Capecitabine

Capecitabine is a precursor of 5-fluoruracil and is approved for the treatment of breast cancer and colorectal cancer [42]. A prospective study of oral capecitabine plus subcutaneous interferon-alfa in four patients with advanced cutaneous SCC showed complete remission in two patients with partial remission in a third patient and the fourth patient dying from unknown causes [60]. A subsequent study with lower-dose capecitabine that is used in colorectal carcinoma in three OTR patients who developed more than one SCC per month showed significant improvement in the development of SCCs, as well as inflammation and regression of clinically apparent premalignant actinic keratoses [61]. Additional studies are needed to measure the utility of this agent in OTRs for the prevention of SCCs and premalignant lesions.

7.4.2.3 Cetuximab

Limited data has also shown that high-risk cutaneous SCC with more than three high-risk features or very high-risk cutaneous SCC displaying lymphovascular, perineural, parotid, periorbital, cartilaginous, or bony invasion; in-transit metastasis; or metastasis that are treated with adjuvant cetuximab in combination with surgery may have improved outcomes [62]. Diffuse alveolar damage that proved fatal, however, has been reported in two lung transplant patients, and cetuximab should therefore not be used in this patient population [63].

7.4.2.4 Sentinel Lymph Node Biopsy

Sentinel lymph node biopsy (SLNB) of truly high-risk tumor cases while not standard of care has also been reported in the literature for surgical staging and may confer further prognostic value [2]. It has been suggested that SLNB may allow for the detection of subclinical nodal involvement with a recent study of SNLB in 24 patients with NMSCs (17 of which were SCC) showing a sensitivity of 88 % and a specificity of 100 % [64]. In this study, Wagner et al. found that seven patients had a tumor-positive node that was not clinically detectible [64]. In a series examining SLNB in SCCs on the trunk and extremities, Reschly et al. found that four of nine patients had positive nodal involvement, with two of these patients dying from metastatic disease within 2 years in comparison to all five of the node-negative patients being alive and well at a mean follow-up of 8 months [65]. Altinyollar et al. studied SNLB and intraoperative lymphatic mapping in 20 patients with SCCs of the lip greater than 2 cm and clinically non-palpable regional lymph nodes showing that three patients (16.6 %) had metastasis of the 90 % of sentinel lymph nodes identified [66]. Two of these three patients with positive sentinel lymph nodes had non-sentinel lymph nodes free of metastasis. Yet, another study by Civantos et al. showed that in 11 cases with high-risk SCC of the skin and four cases of SCC of the lip, only one sentinel lymph node was positive [67]. Still another large study of high-risk head and neck SCC cases found that lesions in proximity to the parotid gland are at significant risk for nodal metastases and should be considered high risk if greater than 4–5 mm in thickness [68]. Given that many high-risk SCCs occur on the head and neck, and the morbidity associated with SLNB especially in the parotid region where the facial nerve must be preserved, this procedure should be in unique high-risk situations, though all patients should have a clinical lymph node examination performed routinely by their physician [2, 14].

7.4.3 Radiotherapy

As mentioned above, radiation therapy as first-line treatment in high-risk SCC should only be considered in inoperable tumors or patients unable to tolerate surgery. Adjuvant radiation therapy has been used in high-risk SCC cases with perineural involvement or in patients with lymph node involvement in order to eradicate microscopic disease that may not have been removed surgically [42]. In a retrospective review of metastatic cutaneous SCC of the head and neck, Veness et al. reported that patients treated with surgery and adjuvant radiation therapy had improved outcomes with a lower rate of recurrence (20 % as compared to 43 % in the surgery-only group) and a higher 5-year disease free survival rate (73 % versus 54 % in the surgery-only group) [69]. The role of radiation therapy in patients with microscopic perineural invasion is controversially reported in the literature, with some studies showing benefit and other studies suggesting good control with surgical excision alone [70]. In general, achievement of a tumor-free plane should be obtained by Mohs migrographic surgery, and patients should be referred to a radiation oncologist for evaluation for adjunctive radiation therapy.

7.5 Other Considerations

OTRs also need more frequent follow-up with their dermatologist or dermatologic surgeon than non-OTRs. Berg and Otley proposed that patients with high-risk SCC be followed every 3 months [2]. Additionally they recommend that those patients with the development of one to four NMSCs per year follow up every 4–6 months, those with the development of 5–10 NMSCs per year follow up every 2–4 months, and those with the development of greater than 10 NMSCs per year follow up every 1–3 months. Data has suggested that the majority of regional metastases occur within 1 year of primary SCC diagnosis and that in-transit metastasis occurs within 10 weeks from initial treatment of the primary SCC making routine and early screening important [21, 49]. Access to dermatology care within transplant centers may improve access to care and awareness of nonmelanoma skin cancers in OTRs [42]. Additionally, organ transplant recipients have also been noted to have poor compliance with sun avoidance and sun protection which have been demonstrated to prevent SCCs and premalignant lesions in this patient population [50, 71].

Finally, decreasing immunosuppression should be considered in life-threatening SCCs or in the case of rapid development of multiple SCCs in this patient population [46]. In a series of six OTRs in whom immunosuppressive medications were stopped due to allograft failure or significant cutaneous malignancy, four had significant reduction in cutaneous carcinogenesis [72]. Such measures, however, are a last effort resort and should only be undertaken in conjunction with the primary transplant physician as altering or decreasing immunosuppressive regimens may result in organ rejection. Additionally, conversion from calcineurin inhibitor to newer treatments such as the mTOR inhibitors should be considered in patients with high-risk and aggressive disease, and while additional studies are needed, this change of therapy may need to take place sooner than current guidelines recommend.

Conclusion

As the field of transplantation has improved, OTRs have become a growing patient population who require increasing consideration from dermatologists and dermatologic surgeons. Increased awareness of the particular nuances of cutaneous malignancy in these patients will contribute to decreased morbidity and mortality. Continued efforts at understanding cutaneous malignancy in this patient population are needed, and further modalities for the treatment and prevention of aggressive cutaneous malignancy must be undertaken. A multidisciplinary approach, with early screening, prevention, and education, is important in the management of these patients. Furthermore, management of precancerous and low-risk SCC with topical or destructive methods, including electrodessication and curettage with imiquimod, 5-FU, and chemoprophylaxis with systemic retinoids, should be considered in all patients to prevent development of high-risk SCCs. Additionally, the use of oral capecitabine and cetuximab have also been suggested in the literature as possibly treatment modalities in these patients though further studies are needed. Finally, adjuvant radiation therapy and sentinel lymph node biopsy should also be considered in select OTR patients with high-risk SCC on a case-by-case basis.

References

1. unos.org [Internet]. [Cited 20 Aug 2013]. Available from: http://unos.org.
2. Berg D, Otley CC. Skin cancer in organ transplant recipients: epidemiology, pathogenesis, and management. J Am Dermatol. 2002;47(1):1–17; quiz 18–20.
3. Carpenter CB. Improving the success of organ transplantation. N Engl J Med. 2000;342(9):647–8.
4. Takemoto SK, Terasaki PI, Gjertson DW, Cecka JM. Twelve years' experience with national sharing of HLA-matched cadaveric kidneys for transplantation. N Engl J Med. 2000;343(15):1078–84.
5. España A, Redondo P, Fernández AL, Zabala M, Herreros J, Llorens R, et al. Skin cancer in heart transplant recipients. J Am Dermatol. 1995;32(3):458–65.
6. Otley CC, Pittelkow MR. Skin cancer in liver transplant recipients. Liver Transpl. 2000;6(3):253–62.
7. Rockville Merkel Cell Carcinoma Group. Merkel cell carcinoma: recent progress and current priorities on etiology, pathogenesis, and clinical management. J Clin Oncol. 2009;27(24):4021–6.
8. Penn I, First MR. Merkel's cell carcinoma in organ recipients: report of 41 cases. Transplantation. 1999;68(11):1717–21.
9. Rüegg CP, Graf N, Mühleisen B, Szucs TD, French LE, Surber C, et al. Squamous cell carcinoma of the skin induces considerable sustained cost of care in organ transplant recipients. J Am Acad Dermatol. 2012;67(6):1242–9.
10. Zwald FO, Brown M. Skin cancer in solid organ transplant recipients: advances in therapy and management: part I. Epidemiology of skin cancer in solid organ transplant recipients. J Am Acad Dermatol. 2011;65(2):253–61; quiz 262.
11. Ulrich C, Kanitakis J, Stockfleth E, Euvrard S. Skin cancer in organ transplant recipients – where do we stand today? Am J Transplant. 2008;8(11):2192–8.
12. Ong CS, Keogh AM, Kossard S, Macdonald PS, Spratt PM. Skin cancer in Australian heart transplant recipients. J Am Dermatol. 1999;40(1):27–34.
13. Veness MJ, Quinn DI, Ong CS, Keogh AM, Macdonald PS, Cooper SG, et al. Aggressive cutaneous malignancies following cardiothoracic transplantation: the Australian experience. Cancer. 1999;85(8):1758–64.
14. Carucci JA. Management of squamous cell carcinoma in organ transplant recipients. Semin Cutan Med Surg. 2003;22(3):177–86.
15. Bordea C, Wojnarowska F, Millard PR, Doll H, Welsh K, Morris PJ. Skin cancers in renal-transplant recipients occur more frequently than previously recognized in a temperate climate. Transplantation. 2004;77(4):574–9.
16. Jensen P, Hansen S, Møller B, Leivestad T, Pfeffer P, Geiran O, et al. Skin cancer in kidney and heart transplant recipients and different long-term immunosuppressive therapy regimens. J Am Dermatol. 1999;40(2 Pt 1):177–86.
17. Jensen P, Møller B, Hansen S. Skin cancer in kidney and heart transplant recipients and different long-term immunosuppressive therapy regimens. J Am Dermatol. 2000;42(2 Pt 1):307.
18. Rowe DE, Carroll RJ, Day CL. Prognostic factors for local recurrence, metastasis, and survival rates in squamous cell carcinoma of the skin, ear, and lip. Implications for treatment modality selection. J Am Dermatol. 1992;26(6):976–90.
19. Sheil AG, Disney AP, Mathew TH, Amiss N. De novo malignancy emerges as a major cause of morbidity

and late failure in renal transplantation. Transplant Proc. 1993;25(1 Pt 2):1383–4.
20. Brantsch KD, Meisner C, Schönfisch B, Trilling B, Wehner-Caroli J, Röcken M, et al. Analysis of risk factors determining prognosis of cutaneous squamous-cell carcinoma: a prospective study. Lancet Oncol. 2008;9(8):713–20.
21. Carucci JA, Martinez JC, Zeitouni NC, Christenson L, Coldiron B, Zweibel S, et al. In-transit metastasis from primary cutaneous squamous cell carcinoma in organ transplant recipients and nonimmunosuppressed patients: clinical characteristics, management, and outcome in a series of 21 patients. Dermatol Surg. 2004;30(4 Pt 2):651–5.
22. Bangash HK, Colegio OR. Management of non-melanoma skin cancer in immunocompromised solid organ transplant recipients. Curr Treat Options Oncol. 2012;13(3):354–76.
23. Patel AA, Swerlick RA, McCall CO. Azathioprine in dermatology: the past, the present, and the future. J Am Acad Dermatol. 2006;55(3):369–89.
24. Perrett CM, Walker SL, O'Donovan P, Warwick J, Harwood CA, Karran P, et al. Azathioprine treatment photosensitizes human skin to ultraviolet A radiation. Br J Dermatol. 2008;159(1):198–204.
25. Flechner SM. Cyclosporine: a new and promising immunosuppressive agent. Urol Clin North Am. 1983;10(2):263–75.
26. Ponticelli C, Tarantino A, Vegeto A. Renal transplantation, past, present and future. J Nephrol. 1999;12 Suppl 2:S105–10.
27. Harvey JJ, East J, Katz FE. Azathioprine-induced lymphocytic neoplasms of NZB mice lack ecotropic murine leukaemia virus. Int J Cancer. 1979;23(2):217–23.
28. Hojo M, Morimoto T, Maluccio M, Asano T, Morimoto K, Lagman M, et al. Cyclosporine induces cancer progression by a cell-autonomous mechanism. Nature. 1999;397(6719):530–4.
29. Karagas MR, Cushing GL, Greenberg ER, Mott LA, Spencer SK, Nierenberg DW. Non-melanoma skin cancers and glucocorticoid therapy. Br J Cancer. 2001;85(5):683–6.
30. Servilla KS, Burnham DK, Daynes RA. Ability of cyclosporine to promote the growth of transplanted ultraviolet radiation-induced tumors in mice. Transplantation. 1987;44(2):291–5.
31. Batiuk TD, Barry JM, Bennett WM, Meyer MM, Tolzman D, Norman DJ. Incidence and type of cancer following the use of OKT3: a single center experience with 557 organ transplants. Transplant Proc. 1993;25(1 Pt 2):1391.
32. Geusau A, Dunkler D, Messeritsch E, Sandor N, Heidler G, Rödler S, et al. Non-melanoma skin cancer and its risk factors in an Austrian population of heart transplant recipients receiving induction therapy. Int J Dermatol. 2008;47(9):918–25.
33. Dantal J, Hourmant M, Cantarovich D, Giral M, Blancho G, Dreno B, et al. Effect of long-term immunosuppression in kidney-graft recipients on cancer incidence: randomised comparison of two cyclosporin regimens. Lancet. 1998;351(9103):623–8.
34. Nabel GJ. A transformed view of cyclosporine. Nature. 1999;397(6719):471–2.
35. Kitchin JE, Pomeranz MK, Pak G, Washenik K, Shupack JL. Rediscovering mycophenolic acid: a review of its mechanism, side effects, and potential uses. J Am Dermatol. 1997;37(3 Pt 1):445–9.
36. Frezza EE, Fung JJ, van Thiel DH. Non-lymphoid cancer after liver transplantation. Hepatogastroenterology. 1997;44(16):1172–81.
37. Duncan FJ, Wulff BC, Tober KL, Ferketich AK, Martin J, Thomas-Ahner JM, et al. Clinically relevant immunosuppressants influence UVB-induced tumor size through effects on inflammation and angiogenesis. Am J Transplant. 2007;7(12):2693–703.
38. Jiang H, Yamamoto S, Nishikawa K, Kato R. Anti-tumor-promoting action of FK506, a potent immunosuppressive agent. Carcinogenesis. 1993;14(1):67–71.
39. Kauffman HM, Cherikh WS, Cheng Y, Hanto DW, Kahan BD. Maintenance immunosuppression with target-of-rapamycin inhibitors is associated with a reduced incidence of de novo malignancies. Transplantation. 2005;80(7):883–9.
40. Campistol JM, Eris J, Oberbauer R, Friend P, Hutchison B, Morales JM, et al. Sirolimus therapy after early cyclosporine withdrawal reduces the risk for cancer in adult renal transplantation. J Am Soc Nephrol. 2006;17(2):581–9.
41. Mathew T, Kreis H, Friend P. Two-year incidence of malignancy in sirolimus-treated renal transplant recipients: results from five multicenter studies. Clin Transplant. 2004;18(4):446–9.
42. Zwald FO, Brown M. Skin cancer in solid organ transplant recipients: advances in therapy and management: part II. Management of skin cancer in solid organ transplant recipients. J Am Acad Dermatol. 2011;65(2):263–79; quiz 280.
43. Mehrany K, Byrd DR, Roenigk RK, Weenig RH, Phillips PK, Nguyen TH, et al. Lymphocytic infiltrates and subclinical epithelial tumor extension in patients with chronic leukemia and solid-organ transplantation. Dermatol Surg. 2003;29(2):129–34.
44. Upjohn E, Bhore R, Taylor RS. Solid organ transplant recipients presenting for Mohs micrographic surgery: a retrospective case–control study. Dermatol Surg. 2012;38(9):1448–55.
45. Brodland DG, Zitelli JA. Surgical margins for excision of primary cutaneous squamous cell carcinoma. J Am Dermatol. 1992;27(2 Pt 1):241–8.
46. Stasko T, Brown MD, Carucci JA, Euvrard S, Johnson TM, Sengelmann RD, et al. Guidelines for the management of squamous cell carcinoma in organ transplant recipients. Dermatol Surg. 2004;30(4 Pt 2):642–50.
47. McCord MW, Mendenhall WM, Parsons JT, Flowers FP. Skin cancer of the head and neck with incidental microscopic perineural invasion. Int J Radiat Oncol Biol Phys. 1999;43(3):591–5.

48. Goldman G. The current status of curettage and electrodesiccation. Dermatol Clin. 2002;20(3):569–78, xi.
49. Martinez JC, Otley CC, Stasko T, Euvrard S, Brown C, Schanbacher CF, et al. Defining the clinical course of metastatic skin cancer in organ transplant recipients: a multicenter collaborative study. Arch Dermatol. 2003;139(3):301–6.
50. Ulrich C, Jürgensen JS, Degen A, Hackethal M, Ulrich M, Patel MJ, et al. Prevention of non-melanoma skin cancer in organ transplant patients by regular use of a sunscreen: a 24 months, prospective, case–control study. Br J Dermatol. 2009;161 Suppl 3:78–84.
51. Ulrich C. Topical treatment of field cancerization. Cancer Treat Res. 2009;146:439–46.
52. Smith KJ, Germain M, Skelton H. Squamous cell carcinoma in situ (Bowen's disease) in renal transplant patients treated with 5 % imiquimod and 5 % 5-fluorouracil therapy. Dermatol Surg. 2001;27(6): 561–4.
53. McNamara IR, Muir J, Galbraith AJ. Acitretin for prophylaxis of cutaneous malignancies after cardiac transplantation. J Heart Lung Transplant. 2002;21(11):1201–5.
54. McKenna DB, Murphy GM. Skin cancer chemoprophylaxis in renal transplant recipients: 5 years of experience using low-dose acitretin. Br J Dermatol. 1999;140(4):656–60.
55. Bavinck JN, Tieben LM, Van der Woude FJ, Tegzess AM, Hermans J, ter Schegget J, et al. Prevention of skin cancer and reduction of keratotic skin lesions during acitretin therapy in renal transplant recipients: a double-blind, placebo-controlled study. J Clin Oncol. 1995;13(8):1933–8.
56. Hoogendijk Akker JM, Harden PN, Hoitsma AJ, Proby CM, Wolterbeek R, Bouwes Bavinck JN, et al. Two-year randomized controlled prospective trial converting treatment of stable renal transplant recipients with cutaneous invasive squamous cell carcinomas to sirolimus. J Clin Oncol. 2013;31(10): 1317–23.
57. Campbell SB, Walker R, Tai SS, Jiang Q, Russ GR. Randomized controlled trial of sirolimus for renal transplant recipients at high risk for nonmelanoma skin cancer. Am J Transplant. 2012;12(5): 1146–56.
58. Euvrard S, Morelon E, Rostaing L, Goffin E, Brocard A, Tromme I, et al. Sirolimus and secondary skin-cancer prevention in kidney transplantation. N Engl J Med. 2012;367(4):329–39.
59. Colegio OR, Hanlon A, Olasz EB, Carucci JA. Sirolimus reduces cutaneous squamous cell carcinomas in transplantation recipients. J Clin Oncol. 2013;31(26):3297–8.
60. Wollina U, Hansel G, Koch A, Köstler E. Oral capecitabine plus subcutaneous interferon alpha in advanced squamous cell carcinoma of the skin. J Cancer Res Clin Oncol. 2005;131(5):300–4.
61. Endrizzi B, Ahmed RL, Ray T, Dudek A, Lee P. Capecitabine to reduce nonmelanoma skin carcinoma burden in solid organ transplant recipients. Dermatol Surg. 2013;39(4):634–45.
62. O'Bryan K, Sherman W, Niedt GW, Taback B, Manolidis S, Wang A, et al. An evolving paradigm for the workup and management of high-risk cutaneous squamous cell carcinoma. J Am Acad Dermatol. 2013;69(4):595–602.
63. Leard LE, Cho BK, Jones KD, Hays SR, Tope WD, Golden JA, et al. Fatal diffuse alveolar damage in two lung transplant patients treated with cetuximab. J Heart Lung Transplant. 2007;26(12):1340–4.
64. Wagner JD, Evdokimow DZ, Weisberger E, Moore D, Chuang T-Y, Wenck S, et al. Sentinel node biopsy for high-risk nonmelanoma cutaneous malignancy. Arch Dermatol. 2004;140(1):75–9.
65. Reschly MJ, Messina JL, Zaulyanov LL, Cruse W, Fenske NA. Utility of sentinel lymphadenectomy in the management of patients with high-risk cutaneous squamous cell carcinoma. Dermatol Surg. 2003;29(2):135–40.
66. Altinyollar H, Berberoğlu U, Celen O. Lymphatic mapping and sentinel lymph node biopsy in squamous cell carcinoma of the lower lip. Eur J Surg Oncol. 2002;28(1):72–4.
67. Civantos FJ, Moffat FL, Goodwin WJ. Lymphatic mapping and sentinel lymphadenectomy for 106 head and neck lesions: contrasts between oral cavity and cutaneous malignancy. Laryngoscope. 2006;112((3 Pt 2 Suppl 109)):1–15.
68. Veness MJ, Palme CE, Morgan GJ. High-risk cutaneous squamous cell carcinoma of the head and neck: results from 266 treated patients with metastatic lymph node disease. Cancer. 2006;106(11):2389–96.
69. Veness MJ, Morgan GJ, Palme CE, Gebski V. Surgery and adjuvant radiotherapy in patients with cutaneous head and neck squamous cell carcinoma metastatic to lymph nodes: combined treatment should be considered best practice. Laryngoscope. 2005;115(5):870–5.
70. Han A, Ratner D. What is the role of adjuvant radiotherapy in the treatment of cutaneous squamous cell carcinoma with perineural invasion? Cancer. 2007;109(6):1053–9.
71. Seukeran DC, Newstead CG, Cunliffe WJ. The compliance of renal transplant recipients with advice about sun protection measures. Br J Dermatol. 1998;138(2):301–3.
72. Otley CC, Coldiron BM, Stasko T, Goldman GD. Decreased skin cancer after cessation of therapy with transplant-associated immunosuppressants. Arch Dermatol. 2001;137(4):459–63.

8 Advances in Management of Merkel Cell Carcinoma in Organ Transplant Recipients: Role of Polyoma Virus and Immunosuppression

Kathryn Serowka, Sarah Arron, and Siegrid S. Yu

Contents

K. Serowka, MD (✉)
Department of Dermatology, University of California – Irvine, Irvine, CA, USA
e-mail: kserowka@uci.edu

S. Arron, MD, PhD • S.S. Yu, MD
Department of Dermatology, University of California, San Francisco, San Francisco, CA, USA
e-mail: arrons@derm.ucsf.edu; yus@derm.ucsf.edu

8.1 Introduction

Merkel cell carcinoma (MCC) is a rare and aggressive primary cutaneous neoplasm. It was first described in 1972 by Toker as a trabecular carcinoma [1]. Since this first description, additional evidence of secretory granules on electron microscopy and neuroendocrine markers, identified with immunohistochemistry, have additionally categorized this tumor as one of neuroendocrine origin.

Although the exact cause of MCC is not precisely known, extensive evidence demonstrates that the immune system is involved with tumor development and progression. The hypothesis of a viral etiology playing a causative role stemmed from this observation and led to the discovery of a new polyomavirus, designated Merkel cell polyomavirus (MCPyV) [2]. Additional investigators have since corroborated the presence of MCPyV in tumor cells and have additionally demonstrated integration of MCPyV DNA into tumor cell DNA [3–7].

Drs. Serowka, Arron, and Yu participated in the drafting of the manuscript and critical revision for important intellectual content. Dr. Serowka has no relevant financial disclosures. Dr. Yu is a paid investigator for Oncosec. Dr. Arron is supported by the National Center for Advancing Translational Sciences, National Institutes of Health, through UCSF-CTSI Grant Number KL2 TR000143. The content of this publication is solely the responsibility of the authors and does not necessarily represent the official views of the NIH.

F. Zwald, M.D. Brown (eds.), *Advances in Transplant Dermatology: Clinical and Practical Implications*, DOI 10.1007/978-3-319-12445-2_8, © Springer International Publishing Switzerland 2015

8.2 Epidemiology

Although MCC remains a rare neoplasm with an incidence of only 0.24 per 100,000 person-years, its incidence rate has tripled since 1986 [8]. The rapidly increasing incidence rate may be partly due to the increased availability of cytokeratin 20 immunohistochemistry, leading to an increased rate of diagnosis [9]. However, this increase may also be attributable to an increase in the highest-risk demographics for MCC: Caucasians over the age of 50 with extensive sun damage and patients with T-cell immunosuppression. The average age of diagnosis is 72, and only five percent of tumors occur in immunocompetent patients under the age of 50 [8, 10, 11].

The immune system plays an important role in MCC tumorigenesis, evidenced by the increased incidence in immunosuppressed patients. The propensity for MCC to arise on sun-damaged skin of elderly Caucasians is likely due to age-related immunosenescence and ultraviolet (UV) radiation–induced cutaneous immunosuppression [8, 10, 12]. Up to 36 % of MCCs occur on the face, the most common anatomical location. Furthermore, the rate of incidence of MCC has been shown to vary regionally with increased rates found in areas with a higher UVB solar index [11]. Recent larger studies of the Surveillance, Epidemiology, and End Results (SEER) database have demonstrated a statistically significant male predominance with 61.5 % of MCCs occurring in men and 38.5 % occurring in women [8, 11].

8.3 Epidemiology of Polyomavirus

Polyomaviruses are non-enveloped double-stranded DNA viruses with a 5kB circular genome. The MCPyV genome consists of an early gene expression region, containing the tumor antigen locus that codes for tumor protein antigen, T antigen, and a late gene expression region that contains genes for capsid and structural proteins. MCPyV, like other human polyoma viruses, is prevalent in most healthy human subjects as measured by serum antibodies to viral capsid proteins [13–15]. Active polyomavirus infection is typically asymptomatic in immunocompetent individuals, but in immunosuppressed renal transplant patients can cause symptomatic disease. For example, in renal transplant recipients, BK polyomavirus can present as nephropathy, and JC polyomavirus can present with progressive multifocal encephalopathy in the setting of HIV infection. Though McPyV does not cause symptomatic acute infection, it is the only polyoma virus that has been shown to integrate into human host genomic DNA. Following primary infection virus is shed continuously from clinically normal skin in the form of assembled virions [16]. Viral DNA has also been detected in respiratory secretions, in anogenital mucosa, and in thc digestive tract, although in lower frequencies [17–19]. Exposure occurs in childhood, as evidenced by 0 % seropositivity in infants, 43 % in children aged 2–5 years old, and 80 % in adults over 50 [13, 14].

Using PCR analysis 64–76 % of MCCs show demonstrable MCPyV [20, 21]. However, MCPyV infection alone is not sufficient to cause carcinogenesis: T antigen truncation, genomic integration, and possibly immunosuppression or loss of specific surveillance for MCPyV antigens are also required [22].

8.4 MCC and Immunosuppression

Up to 10 % of MCCs are found in the setting of decreased immunity. Risk of MCC increases with iatrogenic immunosuppression, HIV infection, and hematologic malignancy. The incidence rate of MCC in immunosuppressed patients is 0.6 per 100,000, a rate that is five- to tenfold greater than the general population [23, 24]. Prolonged systemic immunosuppression predisposes to MCC and is a stage-independent predictor of worsened survival among patients with Merkel cell carcinoma [25].

Chronic lymphocytic leukemia (CLL) and other hematologic malignancies have been associated with an increased incidence and substantially lower overall survival when compared to expected survival of age- and sex-matched patients. Interestingly, the presence of MCPyV has been found in up to 27.1 % of patients with CLL, and in one study all MCCs found in patients with a coexisting diagnosis of CLL tested positive for MCPyV [26, 27]. The risk of MCC is also increased in patients infected with HIV. A majority of the described cases were diagnosed more than 6 months prior to the onset of AIDS, indicating that even moderate immunosuppression can increase the risk for MCC. MCC has also been reported in several patients on TNF-alpha inhibitors [28, 29].

8.5 MCC and Organ Transplantation

OTRs tend to develop MCC at an earlier age and show decreased MCC-specific and overall survival when compared to the general population [25, 30–32] (Fig. 8.1). Average age at diagnosis in OTRs is 53 years, and as many as 29 % of cases may occur in patients under the age of 50 years [30]. Canavan et al. showed that hazard ratios in OTRs are significantly higher than in other types of immunosuppression with a 4-fold increased hazard for progression, 12-fold increased hazard for disease-specific death, and a 10.5-fold increased hazard for overall mortality [33]. The exact mechanism by which iatrogenic immunosuppression worsens the prognosis of MCC is not yet known, but reinstitution of the immune system has reportedly led to regression of MCC in several cases [34, 35].

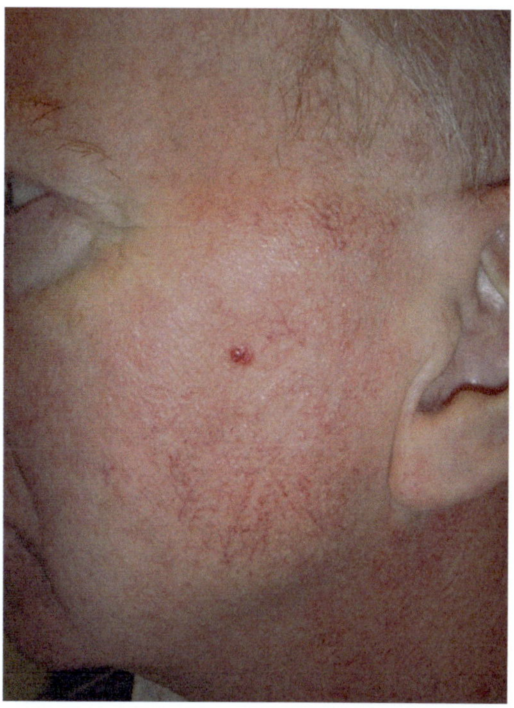

Fig. 8.1 A 56-year-old male 5 years status post renal transplant with 0.4 cm nodule on the left zygomatic cheek

MCC is most likely to occur approximately 6–8 years after transplantation, and the incidence dramatically increases in patients who are greater than 20 years post-transplant [36]. 69 % of post-transplant MCCs occur in male patients partly due to the predominance of men among the OTR population. The majority of MCCs in OTRs, up to 93 % of MCC in OTRs, are diagnosed in renal transplant patients, with heart and liver transplant patients each accounting for approximately 4 % [23].

In three reports involving the withdrawal of immunosuppression in OTRs with MCC, the patients remained disease free for approximately 6 months before developing rapidly progressive disease [34, 37, 38]. In contrast, partial to complete spontaneous regression of MCC in patients without iatrogenic immunosuppression, approximately 20 cases, has also been reported in the literature [34, 39]. Most of these cases occurred soon after a biopsy was performed, likely indicating that trauma stimulated the observed T cell–dominant immune response. In these reports, patients remained disease free decades after regression.

8.6 Clinical Features

The clinical features most commonly associated with MCC are summarized by the mnemonic "AEIOU" and can be used to aid in diagnosis. In tumors that have three or more of the following, a diagnosis of MCC should be suspected: Asymptomatic/nontender, Expanding rapidly, Immunosuppressed, Older than 50 years, and extensive UV damage in a fair-skinned patient. Eighty-nine percent of MCC will have three or more of these features [40].

While MCC most frequently appear on sun-exposed areas, most commonly the head/neck (49 %), followed by the extremities (45 %) and the trunk (15 %) (Fig. 8.2), they can also occur on completely sun-protected areas such as the buttock and vulva [41]. OTRs may have multiple MCCs, and most have other types of skin cancer [23, 30]. The average size at diagnosis in OTRs is 2 cm [42].

8.7 Staging and Prognosis

The American Joint Committee on Cancer (AJCC) MCC staging system was first published in 2010 [43] (Table 8.1). The percentage of patients with localized disease at presentation ranges from 49 to 76 %, with most of the cases of localized disease presenting on the extremities [8, 10, 42].

The relative probability of survival decreases significantly with the finding of regional or meta-

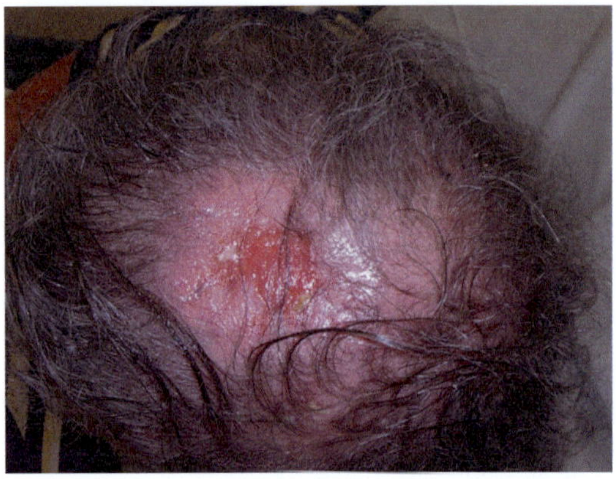

Fig. 8.2 A 66-year-old male 5 years status post bilateral lung transplant with 3.5 cm primary scalp lesion

Table 8.1 AJCC staging system

Tumor	Regional nodes	Distant metastasis
TX – primary tumor cannot be assessed	NX – regional lymph nodes cannot be assessed	M0 – no distant metastasis
T0 – no evidence of primary tumor (e.g., nodal/metastatic presentation without associated primary)	N0 – no regional lymph nodes metastasis	M1 – metastases beyond regional lymph nodes
Tis – in situ primary tumor	cN0 – nodes negative by clinical exam (no pathologic node exam performed)	M1a – metastases to the skin, subcutaneous tissues, or distant lymph nodes
T1 – ≤2 cm maximum tumor dimension	pN0 – nodes negative by pathologic exam	M1b – metastasis to lung
T2 – >2 cm but ≤5 cm maximum tumor dimension	N1 – metastases in regional lymph node(s)	M1c – metastases to all other visceral sites
T3 – >5 cm maximum tumor dimension	N1a – micrometastasis	
T4 – primary tumor invades the bone, muscle, fascia, or cartilage	N1b – macrometastasis N2 – in-transit metastasis	

Stage	T	N	M
0	Tis	N0	M0
IA	T1	pN0	M0
IB	T1	cN0	M0
IIA	T2/T3	pN0	M0
IIB	T2/T3	cN0	M0
IIC	T4	N0	M0
IIIA	Any T	N1a	M0
IIIB	Any T	N1b/N2	M0
IV	Any T	Any N	M1

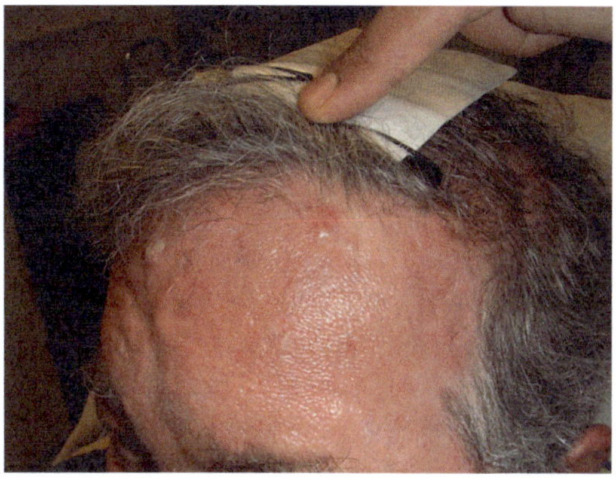

Fig. 8.3 One week after initial diagnosis, a 1 cm biopsy of a left forehead nodule anterior to hairline showing Merkel cell carcinoma

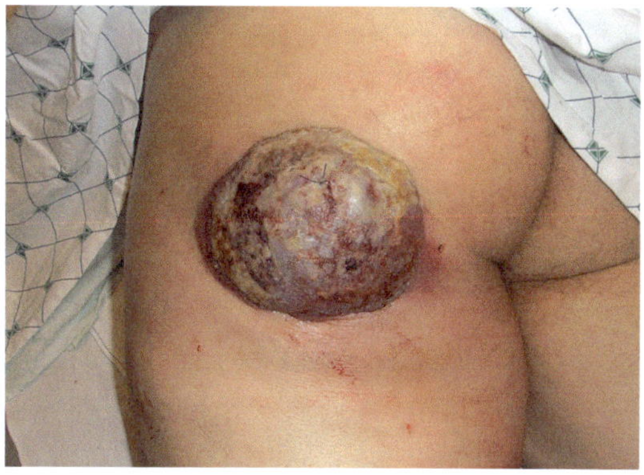

Fig. 8.4 A 59-year-old liver transplant recipient with rapidly enlarging 10 × 13 cm lesion on the left buttock

static spread. MCC patients in the general population who present with local disease have shown a relative survival of 64 % at 5 years, while those with regional nodal disease have a 5-year relative survival that decreases to 39 % (Fig. 8.3). Patients who present with distant metastatic MCC have a dismal 5-year relative survival of only 18 % [44]. Few patients diagnosed with distant metastases survive for 3 years or longer [45]. In OTRs, MCC is even more aggressive than in the general population with 68 % of OTRs presenting with lymph node involvement and 56 % dying from their disease [30].

Additionally improved survival in patients with localized disease can be predicted by size of the tumor, with tumors less than 2 cm showing improved survival [44] (Fig. 8.4). Stage III patients who present with an unknown primary tumor have also been found to have a statistically significant better prognosis compared to Stage III patients with a known primary tumor [46, 47]. It is hypothesized that patients with an unknown primary tumor have most likely undergone spontaneous regression of their primary tumor. This regression may be attributable to a robust immune response and may partially explain their improved survival rates. A robust immune response has been shown in many different ways to improve survival. Detection of high antibody titers of MCPyV was a significant predictor for progression-free survival [48]. Additionally, tumors with a robust CD8+ and CD3+ intratumoral lymphocyte response show greatly better than expected MCC-specific survival [49, 50]. A recent study showed that p63 expression represents a strong risk factor for shortened survival, but this finding has yet to be confirmed by studies on larger cohorts [51].

MCPyV-positive MCCs are less likely to metastasize and have a better prognosis than MCPyV-negative MCCs [52–55]. Additionally, MCPyV-positive tumors have fewer regional nodal metastases at time of diagnosis and are more likely to be located on the extremities than MCPyV DNA–negative MCCs [53]. Differences in tumor biology have been demonstrated and likely account for the differences in outcomes. For example, MCPyV-positive tumors cause carcinogenesis via pRB-mediated oncogenic pathways, while in contrast MCCs with few or no detectable copies of MCPyV depend on alternate oncogenic pathways, such as p53 [52].

Metastases most commonly occur through the lymphatic system, and nodal status is the best predictor of metastatic spread [56]. While distant metastasis is unusual at presentation, eventually as many as 35–50 % of patients will develop distant metastasis. Metastasis is most common to the lymph nodes, skin, lung, brain, bones, and liver [44, 57].

There are currently no evidence-based guidelines recommending how to follow patients for the development of progressive disease. Imaging modalities that have been utilized include (F-18-FDG)-PET scan, CT scan, and radiolabeled octreotide scintigraphy (OctreoScan), though the last is not considered standard of care [58]. FDG-PET has been shown to be better at detecting lymph node [59] and bone metastasis [60] than CT scan; however, it may miss liver metastasis, likely secondary to increased glucose metabolism in the liver, which can be detected with contrast-enhanced diagnostic CT [61]. Paulson et al. demonstrated that serology may be used to detect IgG antibodies to the MCPyV T antigen. These antibodies can be found in 40.5 % of MCC patients and tend to fall rapidly and stay low in patients who do not recur, and increase rapidly prior to detection of disease spread in patients with progression [62]. Additional studies are needed to further evaluate the role of MCPyV T antigen antibodies in monitoring for early signs of recurrent or progressive disease, as a target for future therapeutics.

8.8 Treatment

There remains a significant deficit of randomized control trials to evaluate therapeutic options for MCC. The annually published NCCN guidelines based on best available evidence and consensus recommendations from leading cancer centers can be utilized to guide management. Given the likelihood for an increased incidence and a more aggressive disease course, physicians need to take extra vigilance when caring for OTRs. Patients should have regular full skin and lymph node exams. These exams should be every 3–6 months for the first 2 years after diagnosis and every 6–12 months thereafter. Imaging studies are only needed as clinically indicated. Patients should be educated on performing self-skin examinations on a monthly basis. OTRs have an increased risk of all types of skin cancers, and daily sun protection should be emphasized. A multidisciplinary approach is needed to care for OTRs diagnosed with MCC, as they are likely to have an aggressive disease course. Close follow-up and co-management with the transplant team with possible reduction or revision of immunosuppression may lead to improved outcomes, though no specific data exists.

Currently, treatment is dictated by the clinical stage at presentation and parallels that used in the general population. Wide local excision with 2 cm margins is recommended, followed by histologic examination to confirm clearance of all margins. Margins of at least 2 cm should be obtained whenever possible, as this will decrease the risk for recurrence although it may not improve survival [63–65]. In patients who are not candidates for surgery, radiation can be used to gain local control, and in one report 4 patients who received radiation monotherapy were disease free at 5 years [66].

MCC is a highly radiosensitive tumor. Most studies have demonstrated a positive association between the addition of adjuvant radiation and improved locoregional control [67–72]. While adjuvant radiation may reduce the probability of regional recurrence, it has not been shown to improve overall survival [72].

Lymph node status should be addressed at the time of wide local excision with a sentinel lymph node biopsy (SLNBx). SLNBx has been shown to be a less morbid procedure than full lymphadenectomy and provides significant prognostic information [73, 74]. The histologic status of the SLN can predict the status of the entire lymph node basin that is at risk for metastases [75]. Patients with clinically localized disease and pathologically proven negative nodes have improved survival when compared to those who only undergo clinical nodal evaluation [44]. Patients with a positive SLNBx have been shown to have a three times higher risk of developing recurrent disease than patients with a negative SLNBx, and in one study SLNBx changed the stage of one-third of MCC patients by demonstrating clinically occult microscopic nodal disease, ultimately altering their treatment course [56]. In these patients with clinically node-negative disease, microscopic metastatic disease can take up to 8 months to become clinically apparent [76]. Proper identification and staging of these patients better directs algorithms for treatment of MCC.

Elective lymphadenectomy can be undertaken for treatment of SLN-positive patients and has been associated with improved disease-free survival, but not overall survival [42, 70]. It is important to remember that this procedure comes along with a small but real risk of morbidity including infection, pain, and lymphedema. One large study found that in lymph node–positive disease irradiation to the primary lymph node basin is comparable to surgical outcomes with no detectable difference in overall survival and can be considered as a treatment option in patients with positive lymph nodes [77].

While MCC is generally believed to be a chemotherapy-sensitive neoplasm, no consensus as to chemotherapy treatment regimen exists. Additionally, it is rarely used in the setting of immunosuppression due to increased morbidity/mortality from marrow suppression and sepsis. Agents used to treat MCC are similar to those used to treat small cell lung carcinoma and include platinum-based agents, cyclophosphamide, doxorubicin, vincristine, prednisone, bleomycin, 5-fluorouracil, and various combinations of the above. Most chemotherapeutic regimens provide good initial regression of the lesion; however, recurrences occur commonly within the first 4–15 months following treatment [78]. The benefits of chemotherapy should be weighed against the risks, especially in elderly patients with multiple comorbidities and in immunosuppressed patients. In particular, one retrospective analysis linked patients who received adjuvant chemotherapy to a worse overall survival compared to patients who did not receive chemotherapy [45]. Additionally, there are no established second-line treatments for patients who progress while on chemotherapy. There is a resounding need for novel, biology-driven therapies for this disease.

8.9 Targeted Molecular Therapies

Octreotide, a somatostatin analog, has been shown to have antiproliferative effects on neuroendocrine tumor cells, possibly through the inhibition of tumor angiogenesis (Table 8.2). Because as many as 90 % of MCCs demonstrate somatostatin-2 receptors, octreotide is a promising therapy [79]. Additionally, radiolabeled octreotide scintigraphy may be utilized to detect the presence of these receptors to determine if a patient is likely to have a clinical response. There are two favorable cases reported in the literature of complete remission after somatostatin analog therapy with sustained remissions demonstrated at 10 and 17 months, respectively [80, 81]. Notably, very little toxicity was noted with the use of these medications. Complications reported include carcinoid syndrome and abnormal urinary 5-hydroxy-indoloacetic acid secretion. Disease showed stabilization for at least 6 months (range 1–32 months) [82]. A phase I trial of the somatostatin analog, pasireotide, by the National Institute of Health is currently ongoing.

Pazopanib, a receptor kinase inhibitor that targets both vascular endothelial growth factor

Table 8.2 Targeted molecular therapies

Treatment	Mechanism	Current research	Results
Octreotide	Somatostatin analog	Phase I trial underway with pasireotide by NIH	Median survival time 22 months with disease stabilization of at least 6 months
Pazopanib	Receptor kinase inhibitor – targets VEGF and PDGF receptors	One case report	Complete remission of primary lesion partial remission metastatic lesions; 4 months till progression
YM-155	Downregulates survivin	Mouse xenograft model study	Halted the growth of MCV-positive MCC xenograft tumors and was nontoxic in mice, cytostatic as tumors regrew with withdrawal
PI3K/AKT Inhibitors	Inhibits PI3K and AKT pathways which are upregulated	In vitro studies	Presence of a PIK3CA-activating mutation was associated with sensitivity to treatment in MCC samples with a specific PI3K inhibitor and to a dual PI3K/mTOR inhibitor
Lorvotuzumab Mertansine	Maytansinoid microtubule assembly inhibitor fixed to CD56 monoclonal antibody	Phase I trial complete	2 out of 12 patients with durable complete responses after treatment

(VEGF) and platelet-derived growth factor (PDGF) receptors, has been hypothesized to inhibit tumor growth and angiogenesis. It is currently being used for both renal cell carcinoma and soft tissue sarcoma and is generally well tolerated. There is currently one case report in which a patient with MCC was treated with pazopanib and had complete regression of a scalp tumor and partial regression of pulmonary metastasis. Median time until progression was 4 months. Minimal adverse effects were seen, but dose had to be reduced from 800 mg daily to 400 mg daily after patient developed gallstone pancreatitis [83]. Additionally, a germ line mutation in the PDGFR-α gene that may serve as a marker for potential treatment response has been found in three patients [61].

Survivin is a cellular protein, frequently increased in MCC that is antiapoptotic to tumor cells. YM-155, a small molecule that downregulates survivin, has been found to be effective against other types of cancers in phase I studies and is considered to be safe with a generally low side effect profile [84]. Current studies of YM-155 in a mouse xenograft model of MCC appear promising with halted growth of MCPyV-positive MCC and no toxicity in mice; however, tumor regrowth occurred with withdrawal of the medication indicating it is likely cytostatic and not cytotoxic [85].

MCC has also been shown to be sensitive to PI3K/AKT inhibitors currently in early trials. PI2K/AKT pathway is upregulated in approximately 10 % of MCC tumors and is independent of tumor viral status [86].

Lorvotuzumab mertansine is comprised of a maytansinoid microtubule assembly inhibitor fixed with a humanized monoclonal antibody to CD56. Since CD56 is expressed on almost all MCC, it is hypothesized to target MCC. The phase 1 trial which included 12 MCC patients demonstrated durable complete responses in two of the MCC patients.

8.10 Immunotherapy

The discovery of MCPyV in MCC tumor cells opens the door to new, targeted therapeutic strategies such as immunotherapies (Table 8.3). As viral oncoproteins play a critical role in tumor development of MCPyV-positive MCC, exploiting these oncoproteins and disrupting their function may provide therapeutic benefit. For example, the T antigen–specific N-terminus domain shared by the small and large MCC T antigens may provide a target for vaccine or adoptive T-cell therapies [62]. Furthermore, the presence of viral peptides may be employed to stimulate the immune response against virus-infected tumor cells.

One treatment exploits the upregulation of programmed death-1 (PD-1), an inhibitory cell surface receptor that blocks T-cell receptor (TCR) signaling on lymphocytes. It is commonly upregulated in patients with chronic viral infections and leads to the development of T-cell exhaustion [87]. Additionally, the administration of antibodies to block the interaction of PD-1 with its ligand has been shown to enhance T-cell response. In patients with MCC, PD-1 is upregulated on MCPyV-specific CD8 T cells when compared to control T cells [88]. Clinical trials for efficacy in MCC are currently ongoing. Durable responses have been shown in other tumors and appear to work the best in tumors that express PD-L1 [89]. Because of the immunosuppression and viral nature of many MCC, this is an encouraging therapeutic option.

Ipilimumab is a monoclonal antibody that blocks CTLA-4, an inhibitory receptor found on T cells. By inhibiting the inhibitor, ipilimumab is able to increase T-cell activation. It has been shown to improve survival in metastatic melanoma patients [90, 91] and may have future benefits in the treatment of MCC.

4-1BB is a co-stimulatory receptor expressed on activated T cells that promotes cellular proliferation, survival, and cytokine production. In preclinical studies, 4-1BB agonists have demonstrated ability to activate NF-κB and induce downstream cytokine production, promote leukocyte proliferation, and inhibit tumor growth [92]. A phase I trial is currently underway in patients with advanced/metastatic solid tumors by the NIH.

IL-12 is a cytokine that upregulates the immune system. Additionally, it shifts the

Table 8.3 Immunotherapies

Treatment	Mechanism	Current research	Results
PD-1/PD-1L inhibitors	Blocks TCR signaling on lymphocytes	Phase I clinical trial ongoing	Complete or partial response in non-small cell lung cancer, melanoma, and renal cell cancer; responses lasted 1 year or more in patients with 1 year or more of follow-up
Ipilimumab	Monoclonal antibody blocks CTLA-4 on T cells, increasing T-cell activation	clinical trials underway in MCC	Shown to improve survival in metastatic melanoma, average improved survival 6 months
4-1BB	Co-stimulatory receptor on activated T cells	Phase I trials underway in advanced/metastatic solid tumors	In preclinical trials agonist antibody-activated NF-κB and induce downstream cytokine production, promote leukocyte proliferation, and inhibit tumor growth in a human xenograft tumor model
Intratumoral IL-12+ electroporation	Allows delivery to tumor of IL-12 while avoiding systemic effects; biases towards a TH1 cytokine profile, induces IFN- γ production	Phase I trial in melanoma completed; phase II trials underway in MCC	Complete resolution of distant, nonelectroporated lesions in 10 % of metastatic melanoma; partial or stable response in 42 % and minimal side effects
Systemic interferon (α and β)	Upregulate MHC-1 immune response	Case report – 2 patients	No regression and severe depression in patient 1; progression of all metastasis in patient 2
Intralesional interferon-β	Upregulate MHC-1 immune response	One case report and small-scale trial show local tumor regression	Local tumor regression in injected lesions

immune system towards a TH1 cytokine profile by inducing IFN-γ production by natural killer and T cells. Its use systemically is limited by a temporary immune suppression and toxicity [93]. Due to the limiting toxicities, local administration has been investigated, and ultimately intratumoral injection of a plasmid encoding IL-12 followed by electroporation showed promising immune effects in phase 1 trials using both a melanoma mouse model and human melanoma model. In phase 1 melanoma trials, 10 % of patients showed complete regression of all metastases, and 42 % showed disease stabilization or partial response [94]. Phase II trial for MCC is currently in progress.

MCC has many methods to avoid the immune system, such as downregulating MHC-I, allowing for CD8 T-cell evasion. In fact, more than half of MCC (51 %) demonstrate downregulation of MHC-I. In in vitro MCC cell lines, interferon was able to cause reversal of this MHC-I downregulation [95, 96]. While small-scale trials with systemic interferon (α and β) in patients with MCPyV-positive MCC have thus far been disappointing [97], one case report and a pilot study show successful local tumor regression with intralesional injection of interferon-β [95, 98].

Conclusion

In conclusion, MCC remains an aggressive neoplasm for which we need improved and mechanism-directed therapies. It affects younger organ transplant patients at higher rates than the general population. Additionally, these patients have decreased MCC-specific and overall survival. Additional research is needed into treatment protocols and in the role of reducing/revising immunosuppression for patients with MCC to ultimately improve disease outcomes in OTRs.

Acknowledgement I would like to acknowledge Anna Cogen for her help with this part of the manuscript.

References

1. Toker C. Trabecular carcinoma of the skin. Arch Dermatol. 1972;105(1):107–10.
2. Feng H, et al. Clonal integration of a polyomavirus in human Merkel cell carcinoma. Science. 2008;319(5866):1096–100.
3. Shuda M, et al. T antigen mutations are a human tumor-specific signature for Merkel cell polyomavirus. Proc Natl Acad Sci U S A. 2008;105(42):16272–7.
4. Shuda M, et al. Human Merkel cell polyomavirus infection I. MCV T antigen expression in Merkel cell carcinoma, lymphoid tissues and lymphoid tumors. Int J Cancer. 2009;125(6):1243–9.
5. Foulongne V, et al. Merkel cell polyomavirus and Merkel cell carcinoma, France. Emerg Infect Dis. 2008;14(9):1491–3.
6. Becker JC, et al. MC polyomavirus is frequently present in Merkel cell carcinoma of European patients. J Invest Dermatol. 2009;129(1):248–50.
7. Garneski KM, et al. Merkel cell polyomavirus is more frequently present in North American than Australian Merkel cell carcinoma tumors. J Invest Dermatol. 2009;129(1):246–8.
8. Agelli M, Clegg LX. Epidemiology of primary Merkel cell carcinoma in the United States. J Am Acad Dermatol. 2003;49(5):832–41.
9. Moll I, Kuhn C, Moll R. Cytokeratin 20 is a general marker of cutaneous Merkel cells while certain neuronal proteins are absent. J Invest Dermatol. 1995;104(6):910–5.
10. Albores-Saavedra J, et al. Merkel cell carcinoma demographics, morphology, and survival based on 3870 cases: a population based study. J Cutan Pathol. 2010;37(1):20–7.
11. Miller RW, Rabkin CS. Merkel cell carcinoma and melanoma: etiological similarities and differences. Cancer Epidemiol Biomarkers Prev. 1999;8(2):153–8.
12. O'Connor WJ, Brodland DG. Merkel cell carcinoma. Dermatol Surg. 1996;22(3):262–7.
13. Kean JM, et al. Seroepidemiology of human polyomaviruses. PLoS Pathog. 2009;5(3):e1000363.
14. Tolstov YL, et al. Human Merkel cell polyomavirus infection II. MCV is a common human infection that can be detected by conformational capsid epitope immunoassays. Int J Cancer. 2009;125(6):1250–6.
15. Pastrana DV, et al. Quantitation of human seroresponsiveness to Merkel cell polyomavirus. PLoS Pathog. 2009;5(9):e1000578.
16. Schowalter RM, et al. Merkel cell polyomavirus and two previously unknown polyomaviruses are chronically shed from human skin. Cell Host Microbe. 2010;7(6):509–15.
17. Loyo M, et al. Quantitative detection of Merkel cell virus in human tissues and possible mode of transmission. Int J Cancer. 2010;126(12):2991–6.
18. Kantola K, et al. Merkel cell polyomavirus DNA in tumor-free tonsillar tissues and upper respiratory tract samples: implications for respiratory transmission and latency. J Clin Virol. 2009;45(4):292–5.
19. Babakir-Mina M, et al. Identification of Merkel cell polyomavirus in the lower respiratory tract of Italian patients. J Med Virol. 2010;82(3):505–9.
20. Andres C, et al. Prevalence of MCPyV in Merkel cell carcinoma and non-MCC tumors. J Cutan Pathol. 2010;37(1):28–34.
21. Duncavage EJ, Zehnbauer BA, Pfeifer JD. Prevalence of Merkel cell polyomavirus in Merkel cell carcinoma. Mod Pathol. 2009;22(4):516–21.
22. Chang Y, Moore PS. Merkel cell carcinoma: a virus-induced human cancer. Annu Rev Pathol. 2012;7:123–44.
23. Buell JF, et al. Immunosuppression and Merkel cell cancer. Transplant Proc. 2002;34(5):1780–1.
24. Swann MH, Yoon J. Merkel cell carcinoma. Semin Oncol. 2007;34(1):51–6.
25. Paulson KG, et al. Systemic immune suppression predicts diminished Merkel cell carcinoma-specific survival independent of stage. J Invest Dermatol. 2013;133(3):642–6.
26. Pantulu ND, et al. Detection of a novel truncating Merkel cell polyomavirus large T antigen deletion in chronic lymphocytic leukemia cells. Blood. 2010;116(24):5280–4.
27. Koljonen V, et al. Chronic lymphocytic leukaemia patients have a high risk of Merkel-cell polyomavirus DNA-positive Merkel-cell carcinoma. Br J Cancer. 2009;101(8):1444–7.
28. Krishna SM, Kim CN. Merkel cell carcinoma in a patient treated with adalimumab: case report. Cutis. 2011;87(2):81–4.
29. Linn-Rasker SP, et al. Merkel cell carcinoma during treatment with TNF-alpha inhibitors: coincidence or warning? Ned Tijdschr Geneeskd. 2012;156(22):A4464.
30. Penn I, First MR. Merkel's cell carcinoma in organ recipients: report of 41 cases. Transplantation. 1999;68(11):1717–21.
31. Tarantola TI, et al. Prognostic factors in Merkel cell carcinoma: analysis of 240 cases. J Am Acad Dermatol. 2013;68(3):425–32.
32. Brewer JD, et al. Chronic lymphocytic leukemia is associated with decreased survival of patients with malignant melanoma and Merkel cell carcinoma in a SEER population-based study. J Clin Oncol. 2012;30(8):843–9.
33. Canavan TN, Arron ST, Yu SS. Organ transplant recipients with Merkel cell carcinoma have reduced overall, disease-specific, and progression-free survival independent of stage at presentation. J Invest Dermatol. 2013;133(75):S67.
34. Muirhead R, Ritchie DM. Partial regression of Merkel cell carcinoma in response to withdrawal of azathioprine in an immunosuppression-induced case of metastatic Merkel cell carcinoma. Clin Oncol (R Coll Radiol). 2007;19(1):96.
35. Burack J, Altschuler EL. Sustained remission of metastatic Merkel cell carcinoma with treatment of HIV infection. J R Soc Med. 2003;96(5):238–9.

36. Bordea C, et al. Skin cancers in renal-transplant recipients occur more frequently than previously recognized in a temperate climate. Transplantation. 2004;77(4):574–9.
37. Friedlaender MM, et al. Temporary regression of Merkel cell carcinoma metastases after cessation of cyclosporine. Transplantation. 2002;73(11):1849–50.
38. Plunkett TA, et al. The treatment of Merkel cell carcinoma and its association with immunosuppression. Br J Dermatol. 1998;139(2):345–6.
39. Sais G, Admella C, Soler T. Spontaneous regression in primary cutaneous neuroendocrine (Merkel cell) carcinoma: a rare immune phenomenon? J Eur Acad Dermatol Venereol. 2002;16(1):82–3.
40. Heath M, et al. Clinical characteristics of Merkel cell carcinoma at diagnosis in 195 patients: the AEIOU features. J Am Acad Dermatol. 2008;58(3):375–81.
41. Bottles K, et al. Merkel cell carcinoma of the vulva. Obstet Gynecol. 1984;63(3 Suppl):61S–5.
42. Allen PJ, Zhang ZF, Coit DG. Surgical management of Merkel cell carcinoma. Ann Surg. 1999;229(1):97–105.
43. Edge SB, Compton CC. The American Joint Committee on Cancer: the 7th edition of the AJCC cancer staging manual and the future of TNM. Ann Surg Oncol. 2010;17(6):1471–4.
44. Lemos BD, et al. Pathologic nodal evaluation improves prognostic accuracy in Merkel cell carcinoma: analysis of 5823 cases as the basis of the first consensus staging system. J Am Acad Dermatol. 2010;63(5):751–61.
45. Allen PJ, et al. Merkel cell carcinoma: prognosis and treatment of patients from a single institution. J Clin Oncol. 2005;23(10):2300–9.
46. Chen KT, et al. A better prognosis for Merkel cell carcinoma of unknown primary origin. Am J Surg. 2013;206(5):752–7.
47. Tarantola TI, et al. Unknown primary Merkel cell carcinoma: 23 new cases and a review. J Am Acad Dermatol. 2013;68(3):433–40.
48. Touze A, et al. High levels of antibodies against merkel cell polyomavirus identify a subset of patients with merkel cell carcinoma with better clinical outcome. J Clin Oncol. 2011;29(12):1612–9.
49. Paulson KG, et al. Transcriptome-wide studies of Merkel cell carcinoma and validation of intratumoral CD8+ lymphocyte invasion as an independent predictor of survival. J Clin Oncol. 2011;29(12):1539–46.
50. Sihto H, et al. Tumor infiltrating immune cells and outcome of Merkel cell carcinoma: a population-based study. Clin Cancer Res. 2012;18(10):2872–81.
51. Hall BJ, et al. Immunohistochemical prognostication of Merkel cell carcinoma: p63 expression but not polyomavirus status correlates with outcome. J Cutan Pathol. 2012;39(10):911–7.
52. Bhatia K, et al. Merkel cell carcinoma subgroups by Merkel cell polyomavirus DNA relative abundance and oncogene expression. Int J Cancer. 2010;126(9):2240–6.
53. Sihto H, et al. Clinical factors associated with Merkel cell polyomavirus infection in Merkel cell carcinoma. J Natl Cancer Inst. 2009;101(13):938–45.
54. Sihto H, et al. Merkel cell polyomavirus infection, large T antigen, retinoblastoma protein and outcome in Merkel cell carcinoma. Clin Cancer Res. 2011;17(14):4806–13.
55. Higaki-Mori H, et al. Association of Merkel cell polyomavirus infection with clinicopathological differences in Merkel cell carcinoma. Hum Pathol. 2012;43(12):2282–91.
56. Gupta SG, et al. Sentinel lymph node biopsy for evaluation and treatment of patients with Merkel cell carcinoma: The Dana-Farber experience and meta-analysis of the literature. Arch Dermatol. 2006;142(6):685–90.
57. Pellitteri PK, et al. Merkel cell carcinoma of the head and neck. Head Neck. 2012;34(9):1346–54.
58. Lu Y, et al. Comparison of 18F-FDG PET/CT and 111In pentetreotide scan for detection of Merkel cell carcinoma. Clin Nucl Med. 2012;37(8):759–62.
59. Colgan MB, et al. The predictive value of imaging studies in evaluating regional lymph node involvement in Merkel cell carcinoma. J Am Acad Dermatol. 2012;67(6):1250–6.
60. Hawryluk EB, et al. Positron emission tomography/computed tomography imaging in Merkel cell carcinoma: a study of 270 scans in 97 patients at the Dana-Farber/Brigham and Women's Cancer Center. J Am Acad Dermatol. 2013;68(4):592–9.
61. Miller NJ, et al. Emerging and mechanism-based therapies for recurrent or metastatic Merkel cell carcinoma. Curr Treat Options Oncol. 2013;14(2):249–63.
62. Paulson KG, et al. Antibodies to merkel cell polyomavirus T antigen oncoproteins reflect tumor burden in merkel cell carcinoma patients. Cancer Res. 2010;70(21):8388–97.
63. Hitchcock CL, et al. Neuroendocrine (Merkel cell) carcinoma of the skin. Its natural history, diagnosis, and treatment. Ann Surg. 1988;207(2):201–7.
64. Al-Ghazal SK, et al. Merkel cell carcinoma of the skin. Br J Plast Surg. 1996;49(7):491–6.
65. Queirolo P, et al. Merkel cell carcinoma of the skin. Treatment of primary, recurrent, and metastatic disease: review of clinical cases. Anticancer Res. 1997;17(1B):673–7.
66. Ott MJ, et al. Multimodality management of Merkel cell carcinoma. Arch Surg. 1999;134(4):388–92; discussion 392–3.
67. Veness MJ, et al. Merkel cell carcinoma: improved outcome with adjuvant radiotherapy. ANZ J Surg. 2005;75(5):275–81.
68. Clark JR, et al. Merkel cell carcinoma of the head and neck: is adjuvant radiotherapy necessary? Head Neck. 2007;29(3):249–57.
69. Veness MJ, Morgan GJ, Gebski V. Adjuvant locoregional radiotherapy as best practice in patients with Merkel cell carcinoma of the head and neck. Head Neck. 2005;27(3):208–16.
70. Jabbour J, et al. Merkel cell carcinoma: assessing the effect of wide local excision, lymph node dissection, and radiotherapy on recurrence and survival in early-stage disease–results from a review of 82 consecutive cases diagnosed between 1992 and 2004. Ann Surg Oncol. 2007;14(6):1943–52.

71. Mojica P, Smith D, Ellenhorn JD. Adjuvant radiation therapy is associated with improved survival in Merkel cell carcinoma of the skin. J Clin Oncol. 2007;25(9):1043–7.
72. Jouary T, et al. Adjuvant prophylactic regional radiotherapy versus observation in stage I Merkel cell carcinoma: a multicentric prospective randomized study. Ann Oncol. 2012;23(4):1074–80.
73. Gill G. Sentinel-lymph-node-based management or routine axillary clearance? One-year outcomes of sentinel node biopsy versus axillary clearance (SNAC): a randomized controlled surgical trial. Ann Surg Oncol. 2009;16(2):266–75.
74. Kretschmer L, et al. Postoperative morbidity of lymph node excision for cutaneous melanoma-sentinel lymphonodectomy versus complete regional lymph node dissection. Melanoma Res. 2008;18(1):16–21.
75. Hill ADK, Brady MS, Coit DG. Intraoperative lymphatic mapping and sentinel lymph node biopsy for Merkel cell carcinoma. British Journal of Surgery. 1999;86(4):518–21.
76. Messina JL, et al. Selective lymphadenectomy in patients with Merkel cell (cutaneous neuroendocrine) carcinoma. Ann Surg Oncol. 1997;4(5):389–95.
77. Fang LC, et al. Radiation monotherapy as regional treatment for lymph node-positive Merkel cell carcinoma. Cancer. 2010;116(7):1783–90.
78. Desch L, Kunstfeld R. Merkel cell carcinoma: chemotherapy and emerging new therapeutic options. J Skin Cancer. 2013;2013:327150.
79. Papotti M, et al. Quantitation of somatostatin receptor type 2 in neuroendocrine (Merkel cell) carcinoma of the skin by competitive RT-PCR. Endocr Pathol. 1999;10(1):37–46.
80. Cirillo F, et al. Merkel cell tumor. Report of case and treatment with octreotide. Minerva Chir. 1997;52(11):1359–65.
81. Fakiha M, et al. Remission of Merkel cell tumor after somatostatin analog treatment. J Cancer Res Ther. 2010;6(3):382–4.
82. di Bartolomeo M, et al. Clinical efficacy of octreotide in the treatment of metastatic neuroendocrine tumors. A study by the Italian Trials in Medical Oncology Group. Cancer. 1996;77(2):402–8.
83. Davids MS, et al. Response to a novel multitargeted tyrosine kinase inhibitor pazopanib in metastatic Merkel cell carcinoma. J Clin Oncol. 2009;27(26):e97–100.
84. Tolcher AW, et al. Phase I and pharmacokinetic study of YM155, a small-molecule inhibitor of survivin. J Clin Oncol. 2008;26(32):5198–203.
85. Arora R, et al. Survivin is a therapeutic target in Merkel cell carcinoma. Sci Transl Med. 2012;4(133):133ra56.
86. Nardi V, et al. Activation of PI3K signaling in Merkel cell carcinoma. Clin Cancer Res. 2012;18(5):1227–36.
87. Barber DL, et al. Restoring function in exhausted CD8 T cells during chronic viral infection. Nature. 2006;439(7077):682–7.
88. Afanasiev OK, et al. Merkel polyomavirus-specific T cells fluctuate with Merkel cell carcinoma burden and express therapeutically targetable PD-1 and Tim-3 exhaustion markers. Clin Cancer Res. 2013;19(19):5351–60.
89. Topalian SL, et al. Safety, activity, and immune correlates of anti-PD-1 antibody in cancer. N Engl J Med. 2012;366(26):2443–54.
90. Robert C, et al. Ipilimumab plus dacarbazine for previously untreated metastatic melanoma. N Engl J Med. 2011;364(26):2517–26.
91. Hodi FS, et al. Improved survival with ipilimumab in patients with metastatic melanoma. N Engl J Med. 2010;363(8):711–23.
92. Fisher TS, et al. Targeting of 4-1BB by monoclonal antibody PF-05082566 enhances T-cell function and promotes anti-tumor activity. Cancer Immunol Immunother. 2012;61(10):1721–33.
93. Atkins MB, et al. Phase I evaluation of intravenous recombinant human interleukin 12 in patients with advanced malignancies. Clin Cancer Res. 1997;3(3):409–17.
94. Daud AI, et al. Phase I trial of interleukin-12 plasmid electroporation in patients with metastatic melanoma. J Clin Oncol. 2008;26(36):5896–903.
95. Paulson K, et al. Reversal of local immune evasion mechanisms and regression of human Merkel cell carcinoma by intralesional injection of interferon-beta. J Invest Dermatol. 2011;131:S92.
96. Krasagakis K, et al. Interferon-alpha inhibits proliferation and induces apoptosis of Merkel cell carcinoma in vitro. Cancer Invest. 2008;26(6):562–8.
97. Biver-Dalle C, et al. Use of interferon-alpha in two patients with Merkel cell carcinoma positive for Merkel cell polyomavirus. Acta Oncol. 2011;50(3):479–80.
98. Nakajima H, et al. Screening of the specific polyoma virus as diagnostic and prognostic tools for Merkel cell carcinoma. J Dermatol Sci. 2009;56(3):210–2.

Update in Melanoma in Organ Transplant Patients

9

Ashley Wysong and Seaver L. Soon

Contents

A. Wysong, MD, MS • S.L. Soon, MD (✉)
Dermatology and Dermatologic Surgery, Scripps Clinic, La Jolla, CA, USA
e-mail: awysong@gmail.com; seaversoon@gmail.com

Abbreviations

AJCC	American Joint Committee on Cancer
AKs	Actinic keratosis
FISH	Fluorescent in situ hybridization
HLA	Human leukocyte antigen
IHC	Immunohistochemistry
ITSC	International Transplant Skin Cancer Collaborative
NCCN	National Comprehensive Cancer Network
NIH	National Institutes of Health
NMSC	Nonmelanoma skin cancer
OPTN	Organ Procurement and Transplantation Network
OTRs	Organ transplant recipients
PCR	Polymerase chain reaction
SCOPE	Skin Care in Organ Transplant Patients, Europe
SRTR	Scientific Registry of Transplant Recipients
USA	United States of America

9.1 Introduction

Improvements in human leukocyte antigen (HLA) matching, immunosuppressive regimens, and control of infectious disease have led to a greater number of lifesaving operations for individuals with end-stage organ disease and improved posttransplant graft survival. According to the United States (US) Organ Procurement and Transplantation

F. Zwald, M.D. Brown (eds.), *Advances in Transplant Dermatology: Clinical and Practical Implications*,
DOI 10.1007/978-3-319-12445-2_9, © Springer International Publishing Switzerland 2015

Network (OPTN) and the Scientific Registry of Transplant Recipients (SRTR), approximately 30,000 solid organ transplantations were performed in the USA in 2011. Over 100,000 individuals in the USA receive chronic immunosuppressive therapy to sustain solid organ allografts. These patients are at increased risk of both systemic and cutaneous cancers estimated to be two to four times greater than the general public [27]. The most recent data from the National Institutes of Health (NIH) using a cohort of 175,732 solid OTRs found an overall increased cancer risk with a standardized incidence ratio (SIR) of 2.1 relative to the general population.

The most frequent malignancy in OTRs is skin cancer. Although no US population-based registries exist for nonmelanoma skin cancer (NMSC), the most reliable data to date suggest an approximate 65-fold and 10-fold increase in squamous cell carcinoma and basal cell carcinoma, respectively [11, 14]. The incidence of melanoma is two- to fivefold higher in OTRs than in the general public [14] (OPTN/SRTR 2011 Annual Report). With the rising number of transplanted organs and its attendant risk of melanoma and NMSCs, dermatologists may anticipate caring for an increasing number of transplant recipients. In this chapter, we review the epidemiology, pathogenesis, and management approach to melanoma in transplant recipients and review the three distinct settings in which melanoma may occur in the context of transplantation: (1) melanoma developing prior to transplantation, pretransplant melanoma; (2) melanoma developing after transplantation, posttransplant melanoma; and (3) melanoma transmitted to the recipient from the donor organ, donor-derived melanoma.

9.2 Melanoma in OTRs

9.2.1 Epidemiology

Organ transplant recipients are at increased risk of melanoma due to their chronic state of immunosuppression [1, 12, 21]. Specifically, population-based cohort studies show a 3.4-fold greater risk for melanoma in OTRs in the Netherlands [14] and a standardized incidence ratio of 2.38 (2.14–2.63) for melanoma in OTRs in the USA (OPTN/SRTR 2011 Annual Report) when compared to the general population.

9.2.2 Pathogenesis of Transplant-Associated Melanoma

Melanoma is Otley considered to be an immunogenic tumor, causing immunosuppression in the tumor microenvironment through secretion of anti-inflammatory cytokines, downregulation of major histocompatibility class I antigens on tumor cells, induction of tolerance, and alteration of the typical T-cell response in the host immune system [18]. Specifically, regulatory T cells (CD4+CD25+) are involved in secreting immunosuppressive cytokines and suppressing activation of the antitumor response of the host to melanoma [29]). As such, melanoma is more common in many patient settings associated with immunosuppression, including HIV/AIDS, lymphoma, and the pharmacologic immunosuppression associated with organ transplantation. After receiving transplantation, OTRs require lifelong pharmacologic immunosuppression to prevent potentially fatal organ rejection and loss. The type of immunosuppression and its duration and intensity of use in OTRs are known risk factors for skin cancer, including melanoma. The immunosuppressed state severely reduces immunosurveillance, impairing the normal detection and removal of precancerous or early cancerous lesions. In addition, immunosuppression is believed to aid in the promotion of cancer cell invasiveness and progression [26]. Organ transplant recipients often undergo aggressive induction immunosuppression in the first 3–6 months after transplantation to lower the T-cell response to donor organ antigens and to help avoid acute organ rejection. Following this acute period where the risk of organ loss is the highest, OTRs are placed on maintenance immunosuppression determined by the type of transplanted organ as well as preferences of the transplant team. In the event of life-threatening NMSC or melanoma skin cancer, immunosuppressive regimens are often altered to allow some immune upregulation as a partial treatment strategy. This is particularly the case in melanoma as it is an immunogenic tumor. In fact, several current therapies for melanoma harness the host immune system including IL-2, melanoma vaccines, and CTLA-4 inhibitors such as ipilimumab and PD-1 inhibitor nivolumab.

9.3 Types of Transplant Melanoma

9.3.1 Pretransplant Melanoma

With the growing demand for organ transplantation in the USA, there has been increasing discussion on social equity in organ distribution. To assist in appropriate allocation of organs to recipients with the greatest predicted life expectancy and overall probability of success, OTRs undergo rigorous pretransplant evaluation. Pretransplant comorbidity profiles are reviewed in detail, and a 5-year posttransplant survival probability is estimated for all candidates. In patients with a prior history of invasive melanoma with a quantifiable risk of recurrence, this concept has led to the discussion of what are appropriate pretransplant "wait times" for patients deemed to be at elevated risk for mortality following transplantation.

Traditionally, patients with a prior history of invasive melanoma have been excluded from consideration for organ transplantation or, if listed, given prolonged wait times. There is a paucity of population-based data on patients with pretransplant melanoma, and many of these clinical decisions have been guided in part by data from a few small studies. Specifically, Penn et al. [24] reported recurrent disease and death in 19.4 % of 31 patients with pretransplant melanoma. Disease recurrence occurred between 6 and 30 months posttransplant, leading the authors to recommend a 5-year wait period until transplantation for "most melanoma" and 2 years for "very thin" melanoma. However, growing evidence suggests that a history of invasive melanoma may not be associated with increased recurrence or mortality risk after transplantation.

Recent studies suggest that there is no statistically significant increase in recurrence or mortality in patients with a history of malignant melanoma [7]. The Skin Care in Organ Transplant Patients, Europe (SCOPE) cohort found no melanoma recurrences or melanoma-related deaths in patients with a pretransplant melanoma after 60-month follow-up ($n=9$) [17] posttransplantation. Similarly, a retrospective case series from Mayo Clinic followed 12 patients with pretransplant melanoma from 1978 to 2007 with no recurrences and 100 % 2-year melanoma-specific survival on an average follow-up of 3.5 years; the majority (90 %) were in situ or stage I melanoma [8]. Of note, these outcomes followed a median wait time between melanoma diagnosis and transplant of 7.8 and 3.8 years for the SCOPE and Mayo cohorts, respectively. Finally, Brewer et al. [5] found no recurrence and 100 % 10-year melanoma-specific survival in 17 patients with a history of melanoma and a median wait time of 10 years between melanoma diagnosis and transplantation. In aggregate, these data suggest that a pretransplant history of melanoma may not be an absolute contraindication to organ transplantation.

9.3.2 Posttransplant Melanoma

The incidence of de novo malignant melanoma developing in OTRs after transplantation is estimated to be three to five times higher than the general public [10]. The most recent data from the US Scientific Registry of Transplant Recipients analyzing 175,732 solid OTR showed a standardized incidence ratio of 2.38 relative to the general population [9]. Of note, African-Americans with renal transplants were found to have an annual incidence of melanoma 17.2 times greater than the general African-American population [12].

The risk factors for developing melanoma in OTRs appear to be similar to those in the general population, including a history of dysplastic nevi, blistering sunburns, other skin cancers, and a family history of melanoma [8, 15]. In the SCOPE cohort, 67 % of OTRs with posttransplant melanoma were found to have intermediate or high cumulative sun exposure [17]. In addition, posttransplantation melanoma risk appears to be associated with an older age at the time of transplantation [12] and male gender [24]. The reported mean time to diagnosis is 5–11 years [5, 8, 10, 15]. The most common anatomic sites are the trunk, arms, and shoulders [8, 15], followed by the head and neck [24].

As expected, the prognosis of posttransplant melanoma in OTRs has been reported to be worse than that of the general population, with the most marked differences observed in those with a greater Breslow thickness. In 2011, Brewer et al. reported a 51 % 3-year survival in OTRs with a Breslow depth of 1.51–3.0 mm compared to the expected 87 % survival in SEER controls. In this study, subgroup analysis suggested a significantly higher melanoma-specific mortality in cardiac transplant patients, who typically take higher doses of immunosuppressants, with Breslow thickness greater than 1.51 mm. These findings highlight the effect of the level of immunosuppression in the prognosis of melanoma. In the SCOPE data [17], the overall melanoma-specific mortality rate in 91 OTRs with posttransplant melanoma was 13 % (11/85) with a significantly worse prognosis for stage T3 and T4 posttransplant melanomas (HR 11.49 (3.59–36.82)). In contrast, the Mayo Clinic review of 48 melanomas in 43 OTRs from 1978 to 2007 showed outcomes in immunosuppressed transplant recipients ($n=31$) to be similar to prognostically matched non-immunosuppressed patients. Of note, the authors noted that the small number of cases limited statistical comparisons.

In regard to treatment of posttransplant melanoma, it should generally parallel the workup and treatment of melanoma in the non-transplant population. Newly diagnosed melanoma should undergo wide local excision with the depth of invasion determining surgical margins and need for sentinel lymph node biopsy per American Joint Committee on Cancer (AJCC) and National Comprehensive Cancer Network (NCCN) clinical practice guidelines.

In the event of lymph node involvement, it has been suggested that an expert consensus (i.e., Institutional Tumor Board) should be sought as well as a more aggressive treatment approach including the consideration of lymphadenectomy, adjuvant therapies, and a reduction or discontinuation of immunosuppression. The International Transplant Skin Cancer Collaborative (ITSCC) and SCOPE have both outlined specific recommendations for a reduction in immunosuppression in patients with numerous or life-threatening skin cancers based on the stage and type of skin cancer as well as the type of donor organ [23]. Recommendations for the level of reduction in immunosuppression (mild, moderate, and severe) are based on the stage of melanoma and on the type of organ transplanted. In general, the reduction of immunosuppression is more aggressive for higher stages of melanoma and in renal transplant patients, compared to other organs, as dialysis is a safe alternative in the setting of organ failure or rejection. While sirolimus has been shown to have antitumor effects through inhibition of mTOR and a reduction of SCCs in OTRs (citation), similar findings have not been seen in melanoma. Nonetheless, some transplant teams recommend the addition of an mTOR inhibitor when adjusting immunosuppressive regimens in the setting of posttransplant melanoma. In general, all changes in immunosuppressive regimens should be made as part of multidisciplinary care team including oncology, transplantation surgery and medicine, and dermatology.

Close collaboration by dermatologists with the transplant team throughout the process is paramount, particularly surrounding ongoing skin cancer screening and changes in immunotherapy in the event of numerous or life-threatening skin cancers. A dermatologic follow-up strategy of OTRs has been suggested by Berg and Otley (2002) [3] including an initial dermatologic consultation followed by annual examination by transplant physicians in those without a history of skin cancer or actinic keratosis (AKs) until skin lesions arise. A transplant dermatologist should see OTRs with a history of AKs or NMSC every 6 months posttransplant. OTRs with a history of multiple NMSC and a high-risk SCC or melanoma should be seen every 2–3 months. Visits should include thorough whole body skin examinations as well as extensive sun protection counseling.

9.3.2.1 Donor-Derived Melanoma: Transmission to OTRs

Reports of cancer being transmitted to transplant recipients through the donor organ itself date back to the first reported homologous transplant of a metastatic melanoma lesion in 1965 [16, 25]. As discussed in the immunology section, the immunosuppressed milieu presents an ideal setting for the development or advancement of malignancy. While donor-derived malignancy is rare in OTRs, melanoma has been reported to be the most commonly transmitted tumor-causing distant metastasis [24]. A population-based study by Birkeland and Storm [4] suggests that overall risk of transmission of a donor-derived malignancy is around 0.2 % with a 1.3 % risk of having a donor with an undetected malignancy. The largest case series of donor-derived melanoma reported 13 donors transmitting melanoma to 75 % (21 of 28) of recipients. A recent review by Zwald et al. [33] combined all case reports and case series to date of donor-derived melanoma with 17 donors providing organs to 44 recipients, 80 % of whom (35/44) developed melanoma. Typically, these OTRs developed melanoma within several months to 3 years following the transplantation.

As the melanoma-specific death rate and 5 year survival rate from donor-derived melanoma have been reported to be approximately 65 % [20, 33] and 5 % [17], respectively, the use of additional screening techniques in donor selection may be warranted. In the case series of allogeneic melanomas reported by Penn et al. [24], of 11 donors, 4 had a previous diagnosis of melanoma and the majority (55 %) were misdiagnosed with primary brain tumors or cerebrovascular accidents which were presumably metastatic melanoma to the brain. These findings call for the need for an increased index of suspicion in all potential donors with a personal or family history of melanoma, a history of multiple excised moles, or unknown cerebral neoplasm as the cause of death. Some suggest that a prior history of melanoma, even if fully excised and disease-free for several years, should be a contraindication for organ donation given the possibility of latent melanoma or late recurrence. One report of donor transmission of malignant melanoma to a lung transplant recipient occurred 32 years after curative resection of the donor's melanoma [2]. In addition, the use of sophisticated screening techniques of donor organs such as PCR-based microsatellite markers, immunohistochemistry (IHC), DNA typing, and FISH as appropriate to determine if the tumor in the recipient is of donor origin [20].

Once donor-derived melanoma is identified in OTRs, there are no guidelines and little data to support the appropriate treatment. In the case of kidney transplant recipients, most transplant physicians support withdrawal of immunosuppression based on anecdotal reports of host immunologic rejection of both the allogeneic organ and the tumor [23, 30, 31]. This is typically followed by donor organ removal and consideration of re-transplantation after a significant disease-free period. Although an option for renal transplant recipients, this strategy is impractical in most other solid organ transplant recipients – heart, lung, liver, and bowel – as there are fewer options for substitute organ support. In these cases, a reduction in immunosuppression may be helpful, particularly in those individuals with a greater degree of antigen mismatch between the allogeneic tumor and the recipient. If a reduction of immunosuppression is not successful, therapies such as interferon, tumor vaccines, and lymphokine-activated killer cells have been reported to help boost the immune response [28]. In addition, a recent report showed a complete response of donor-derived melanoma to anti-CTLA4 inhibitor, ipilimumab [6].

9.4 Summary

When evaluating and treating melanoma in transplant patients, it is helpful to think of the three categories of transplant melanoma: pretransplant, posttransplant, and donor-derived melanoma. Dermatologists should be closely involved in optimizing skin health and melanoma care throughout the transplant process. Initially, dermatologists can screen transplant candidates to help identify a history of pretransplant melanoma or atypical/dysplastic nevi, family history of melanoma, extensive cumulative sun exposure, and other high-risk factors for posttransplant melanoma. For those with a history of pretransplant melanoma, AJCC melanoma staging should help guide wait times prior to transplantation to ensure ethical allocation of a scarce resource. In addition, OTRs should continue to receive extensive education regarding the increased skin cancer risk and need for skin self-examination, sunscreen use, and other sun avoidance behaviors posttransplant. This is particularly important as studies have shown that patients with access to a specialist transplant dermatologist and who have undergone pretransplant counseling have a higher rate of sunscreen use posttransplant [13, 19]. Finally, while donor-derived melanoma is rare in OTRs, it has been reported as the most commonly transmitted tumor-causing distant metastasis and is associated with a poor overall survival. An increased index of suspicion is warranted in all potential donors with a personal or family history of melanoma, a history of multiple excised moles, or unknown cerebral neoplasm as the cause of death.

References

1. Ali FR, Lear JT. Melanoma in organ transplant recipients: incidence, outcomes, and management considerations. J Skin Cancer. 2012, epub.
2. Bajaj NS, Watt C, Hadjiliadis D, et al. Donor transmission of malignant melanoma in a lung transplant recipient 32 years after curative resection. Transpl Int. 2010;23(7):e26–31.
3. Berg, Otley. The reference is Skin cancer in organ transplant recipients. Epidemiology, pathogenesis and management. J Am Acad Dermatol. 2002;47(1): 1–17.
4. Birkeland SA, Storm HH. Risks for tumor and other disease transmission by transplantation: a population-based study of unrecognized malignancies and other diseases in organ donors. Transplantation. 2002;74: 1409–13.
5. Brewer JD, Christenson LJ, Weaver AL, et al. Malignant melanoma in solid transplant recipients: collection of database cases and comparison with surveillance, epidemiology, and end results data for outcome analysis. Arch Dermatol. 2011;147(7):790–6.
6. Chen KT, Olszanski A, Farma JM. Donor transmission of melanoma following renal transplant. Case Rep Transplant epub 2012. http://dx.doi.org/10.1155/2012/764019.
7. Colegio OR, Proby CM, Bordeaux JS, McGregor JM, Melanoma Working Group of the International Transplant Skin Cancer C, Skin Care in Organ Transplant Patients E. Prognosis of pretransplant melanoma. Am J Transplant. 2009;9(4):862.
8. Dapprich DC, Weenig RH, Rohlinger AL, Weaver AL, et al. Outcomes of melanoma in recipients of solid organ transplantation. J Am Acad Dermatol. 2008;59:405–17.
9. Engels EA, Pfeiffer RM, Fraumeni JF, Kasiske BL, et al. Spectrum of cancer risk among US solid organ transplant recipients: the transplant cancer match study. JAMA. 2011;306(17):1891–901.
10. Euvrard S, Kanitakis J, Claudy A. Skin cancers after organ transplantation. N Engl J Med. 2003;348:1681–91.
11. Hartevelt MM, Bavenick JN, Kootte AM, Vermeer BJ, Vandenbroucke JP. Incidence of skin cancer after renal transplantation in the Netherlands. Transplantation. 1990;49:506–9.
12. Hollenbeak CS, Todd MM, Billingsley EM, et al. Increased incidence of melanoma in renal transplant recipients. Cancer. 2004;104:1962–7.
13. Ismail F, Mitchell L, Casabonne D, et al. Specialist dermatology clinics for organ transplant recipients significantly improve compliance with photoprotection and levels of skin cancer awareness. Br J Dermatol. 2006;155:916–25.
14. Jensen P, Hansen S, Moller B, Leivestad T, Pfefer P, et al. Skin cancer in kidney and heart transplant recipients and different long-term immunosuppressive therapy regimens. J Am Acad Dermatol. 1999;40:177–86.
15. Le Mire L, Hollowood K, Gray D, et al. Melanomas in renal transplant recipients. Br J Dermatol. 2006; 154(3):472–7.
16. Martin DC, Rubini M, Rosen VJ. Cadaveric renal homotransplantations with inadvertent transplantation of cancer. JAMA. 1965;192:32.
17. Matin RN, Mesher D, Proby CM, McGregor JM, et al. Melanoma in organ transplant recipients: clinicopathological features and outcome in 100 cases. Am J Transplant. 2008;8:1891–900.
18. McCarter MD, Baumgartner J, Escobar GA, et al. Immunosuppressive dendritic and regulatory T cells are upregulated in melanoma patients. Ann Surg Oncol. 2007;14(10):2854–60.
19. Mihalis EL, Wysong A, Boscardin WJ, et al. Factors affecting sunscreen use and sun avoidance in a US national sample of organ transplant recipients. Br J Dermatol. 2013;168(2):346–53.
20. Morris-Stiff G, Steel A, Savage P, Devlin J, et al. Transmission of donor melanoma to multiple organ transplant recipients. Am J Transplant. 2004;4:444–6.

21. Multigonda T, Levender MM, O'Neill JL, West CE, et al. Incidence, risk factors, and preventative management of skin cancers in organ transplant recipients: a review of single and multicenter retrospective studies from 2006 to 2010. Dermatol Surg. 2013; 39:345–64.
22. Organ Procurement and Transplantation Network and the Scientific Registry of Transplant Recipients: OPTN/SRTR 2011 Annual Data Report. Rockville: Department of Health and Human Services, Health Resources and Services Administration, Healthcare Systems Bureau, Division of Transplantation; 2012.
23. Otley CC, Berg D, Ulrich C, et al. Reduction of immunosuppression for transplant-associated skin cancer: expert consensus survey. Br J Dermatol. 2006;154(3):395–400.
24. Penn I. Malignant melanoma in organ allograft recipients. Transplantation. 1996;61:274–8.
25. Scanlon EF, Hawkins RA, Fox WW, Smith WS. Fatal homotransplanted melanoma: a case report. Cancer. 1965;13:782–9.
26. Servilla KS, Burnham DK, Daynes RA. Ability of cyclosporine to promote the growth of transplanted ultraviolet radiation-induced tumors in mice. Transplantation. 1987;44:291–5.
27. Sheil AG. Development of malignancy following renal transplantation in Australia and New Zealand. Transplant Proc. 1992;24:1275–9.
28. Suranyi MG, Hogan PG, Falk MC, et al. Advanced donor-origin melanoma in a renal transplant patient. Transplantation. 1998;66:655.
29. Viguier M, Lemaitre F, Verola O, et al. Foxp3 expressing CD4+CD25+ regulatory T cells are overrepresented in human metastatic melanoma lymph nodes and inhibit the function of infiltrating T cells. J Immunol. 2004;173(2):1444–53.
30. Wilson RN, Hager EB, Hampers CL, et al. Immunologic rejection of human cancer transplanted with a renal allograft. N Engl J Med. 1968;278:479.
31. Younis FM, Fernando ON, Sweny P, et al. Malignant melanoma in a patient with a renal transplant. Lancet. 1980;2:1141.
32. Zwald FO, Christenson LJ, Billingsley EM, et al. Melanoma in solid organ transplant recipients. Am J Transplant. 2010;10(5):1297–304.

MIX
Papier aus verantwortungsvollen Quellen
Paper from responsible sources
FSC® C105338

If you have any concerns about our products,
you can contact us on
ProductSafety@springernature.com

In case Publisher is established outside the EU,
the EU authorized representative is:
Springer Nature Customer Service Center GmbH
Europaplatz 3, 69115 Heidelberg, Germany

Printed by Libri Plureos GmbH
in Hamburg, Germany